STUDY GUIDE *for*

MEMMLER'S
Structure and Function of the Human Body

10TH EDITION

Kerry L. Hull

Professor
Department of Biology
Bishops's University
Sherbrooke, Quebec
Canada

Barbara Janson Cohen

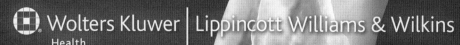

Wolters Kluwer | Lippincott Williams & Wilkins

Health

Philadelphia · Baltimore · New York · London
Buenos Aires · Hong Kong · Sydney · Tokyo

Executive Editor: David Troy
Senior Product Manager: Eve Malakoff-Klein
Designer: Terry Mallon
Artist: Christine Vernon/Hearthside and Dragonfly Media Group
Cover Image: Imagineering
Compositor: SPi Global
Printer: C&C Offset Printing

10th Edition

Library of Congress Cataloging-in-Publication Data on file

ISBN 978-1-6091-3901-8

Care has been taken to confirm the accuracy of the information present and to describe generally accepted practices. However, the authors, editors, and publisher are not responsible for errors or omissions or for any consequences from application of the information in this book and make no warranty, expressed or implied, with respect to the currency, completeness, or accuracy of the contents of the publication. Application of this information in a particular situation remains the professional responsibility of the practitioner; the clinical treatments described and recommended may not be considered absolute and universal recommendations.

The authors, editors, and publisher have exerted every effort to ensure that drug selection and dosage set forth in this text are in accordance with the current recommendations and practice at the time of publication. However, in view of ongoing research, changes in government regulations, and the constant flow of information relating to drug therapy and drug reactions, the reader is urged to check the package insert for each drug for any change in indications and dosage and for added warnings and precautions. This is particularly important when the recommended agent is a new or infrequently employed drug.

Some drugs and medical devices presented in this publication have Food and Drug Administration (FDA) clearance for limited use in restricted research settings. It is the responsibility of the health care providers to ascertain the FDA status of each drug or device planned for use in their clinical practice.

To purchase additional copies of this book, call our customer service department at (800) 638-3030 or fax orders to (301) 223-2320. International customers should call (301) 223-2300.

Visit Lippincott Williams & Wilkins on the Internet: http://www.lww.com. Lippincott Williams & Wilkins customer service representatives are available from 8:30 am to 6:00 pm, EST.

9 8 7 6 5 4 3 2 1

The *Study Guide for Memmler's Structure and Function of the Human Body*, 10th edition, helps students learn foundational concepts in anatomy and physiology required for success in allied health occupations. Although it will be more effective when used in conjunction with the 10th edition of *Memmler's Structure and Function of the Human Body*, the *Study Guide* may also be used to supplement other textbooks on basic anatomy and physiology. The questions in this edition reflect revisions and updating of the text. The labeling and coloring exercises are taken from the illustrations designed for the book.

The exercises are designed to facilitate student learning, not merely to test knowledge. Each chapter contains three main components. The first section, "Addressing the Learning Outcomes," can be completed as students read through the chapter. It contains exercises in many formats, including labeling, coloring, matching, and short answer, all designed to foster active learning. The second section, "Making the Connections," asks students to complete a concept map integrating information from multiple learning outcomes. Finally, "Testing Your Knowledge" includes multiple choice, true/false, completion, short answer, and essay questions to identify areas requiring further study. Within this section, "Practical Applications" questions use everyday situations to test students' understanding of a subject.

All answers to the *Study Guide* questions are in the *Instructor's Manual* that accompanies the text.

Learning about the Human Body

You already have some ideas about the human body that will influence how you learn the information in this textbook. Many of your theories are correct, and this *Study Guide*, created to accompany the 10th edition of *Memmler's Structure and Function of the Human Body*, will simply add detail and complexity to these ideas. Other theories, however, may be too simplistic. It can be difficult to replace these ingrained beliefs with more accurate information. For instance, many students think that the lungs actively inflate and deflate as we breathe, but it is the diaphragm and the rib-cage muscles that accomplish all of the work. Learning physiology or any other subject therefore involves:

1. **Construction**: Adding to and enhancing your previous store of ideas.
2. **Reconstruction**: Replacing misconceptions (prior views and ideas) with scientifically sound principles.
3. **Self-monitoring**. Construction and reconstruction require that you also monitor your personal understanding of a particular topic and consciously formulate links between what you are learning and what you have previously learned. Rote learning is not an effective way to learn anatomy and physiology (or almost anything else, for that matter). **Metacognition** is monitoring your own understanding. Metacognition is very effective if it takes the form of self-questioning during the lectures. Try to ask yourself questions during lectures, such as "What is the prof trying to show here?" "What do these numbers really mean?" or "How does this stuff relate to the stuff we covered yesterday?" Self-questioning will help you create links between concepts. In other words, try to be an active learner during the lectures. Familiarity with the material is not enough. You have to internalize it and apply it to succeed. You can greatly enhance your ability to be an active learner by reading the appropriate sections of the textbook before the lecture.

Each field in biology has its own language. This language is not designed to make your life difficult; the terms often represent complex concepts. Rote memorization of definitions will not help you learn. Indeed, because biological terms often have different meanings in everyday conversation, you probably hold some definitions that are misleading and must be revised. For example, you may say that someone has a "good metabolism" if they can eat enormous meals and stay slender. However, the term "metabolism" actually refers to all of the chemical reactions that occur in the body, including those that build muscle and fat. We learn a new language not by reading about it but by using it. The *Study Guide* you hold in your hands employs a number of learning techniques in every chapter to help you become comfortable with the language of anatomy and physiology.

Addressing the Learning Outcomes

The exercises in this section will help you master the material both verbally and visually. Work through the section as you read the textbook chapter—completing the exercises will help you actively learn the material, improving your chances of remembering it at exam time.

The labeling and coloring exercises will be especially useful for mastering anatomy. You can use these exercises in two ways. First, follow the instructions to label and color (when appropriate) the diagram, using your textbook if necessary. Second, use the diagrams for exam preparation by covering up the label names and practicing naming each structure. Coloring exercises are fun and have been shown to enhance learning.

"Making the Connections": Learning through Concept Maps

This learning activity uses concept mapping to master definitions and concepts. You can think of concept mapping as creating a web of information. Individual terms have a tendency to get lost, but a web of terms is more easily maintained in memory. You can make a concept map by following these steps:

1. Select the concepts to map (6–10 is a good number). Try to use a mixture of nouns, verbs, and processes.
2. If one exists, place the most general, important, or overriding concept at the top or in the center and arrange the other terms around it. Organize the terms so that closely related terms are close together.
3. Draw arrows between concepts that are related. Write a sentence to connect the two concepts that begins with the term at the beginning of the arrow and ends with the term at the end of the arrow.

For instance, consider a simple concept map composed of three terms: student learning, professors, and textbooks. Write the three terms at the three corners of a triangle, separated from each other by 3 to 4 inches. Next is the difficult part: devising connecting phrases that explain the relationship between any two terms. What is the essence of the relationship between student learning and professors? An arrow could be drawn from professors to student learning, with the connecting phrase "*can explain difficult concepts to facilitate.*" The relationship would be "*Professors **can explain difficult concepts to facilitate** student learning.*" Draw arrows between all other term pairs (*student learning* and *textbooks*, *textbooks* and *professors*) and try to come up with connecting phrases. Make sure that the phrase is read in the direction of the arrow.

    There are two concept mapping exercises for most chapters. The first exercise consists of filling in boxes and, in the later maps, connecting phrases. The guided concept maps for Chapters 1 through 6 ask you to think of the appropriate term for each box. The guided concept maps for Chapters 7 through 21 are more traditional concept maps. Pairs of terms are linked together by a connecting phrase. The phrase is read in the direction of the arrow. For instance, an arrow leading from "*genes*" to "*chromosomes*" could result in the phrase "*Genes **are found on pieces of DNA called** chromosomes.*" The second optional exercise provides a suggested list of terms to use to construct your own map. This second exercise is a powerful learning tool, because you will identify your own links between concepts. The act of creating a concept map is an effective way to understand terms and concepts.

Testing Your Knowledge

These questions should be completed after you have read the textbook and completed the other learning activities in the study guide. Try to answer as many questions as possible without referring to your notes or the text. As in the end-of-chapter questions, there are three different levels of questions. Type I questions (Building Understanding) test simple recall: how well have you learned the material? Type II questions (Understanding Concepts) examine your ability to integrate and apply the information in simple practical situations. Type III questions (Conceptual Thinking) are the most challenging. They ask you to apply your knowledge to new situations and concepts. There is often more than one right answer to Conceptual Thinking questions. The answers to all questions are available from your instructor.

Learning from the World Around You

The best way to learn anatomy and physiology is to immerse yourself in the subject. Tell your friends and family what you are learning. Discover more about recent health advances from television, newspapers, magazines, and the Internet. Our knowledge about the human body is constantly changing. The work you will do using the *Study Guide* can serve as a basis for lifelong learning about the human body.

Contents

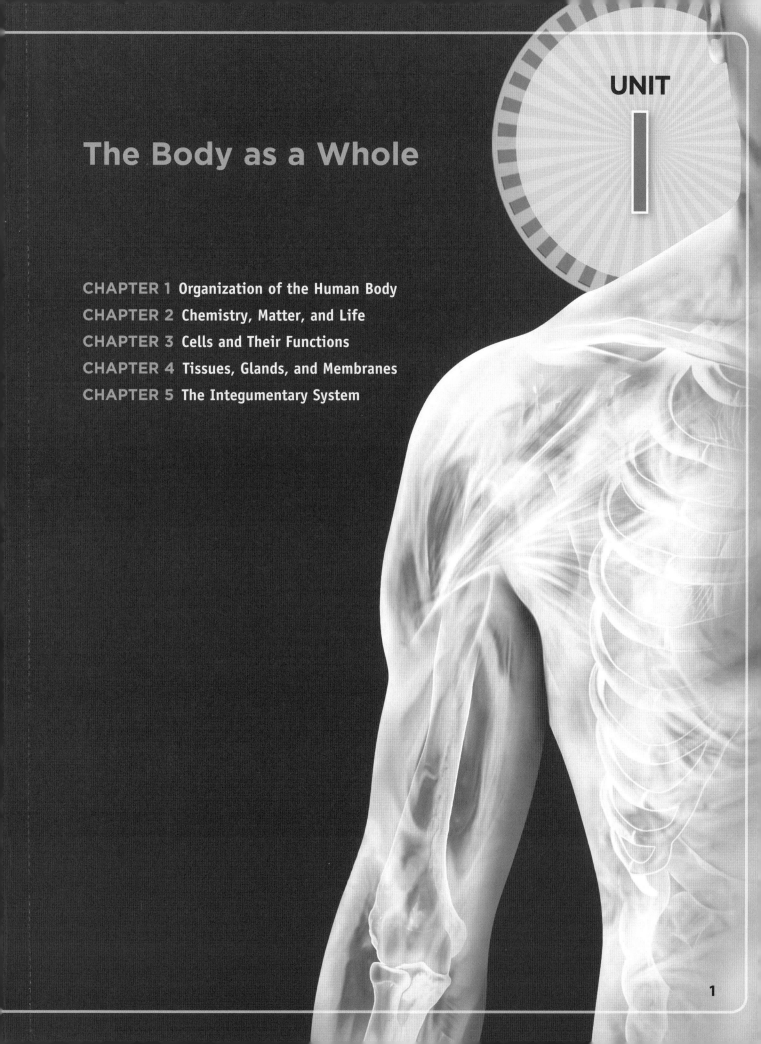

The Body as a Whole

CHAPTER

1

Organization of the Human Body

Overview

Anatomy is the study of body structure, whereas **physiology** is the study of how the body functions.

Living things are organized from simple to complex levels. The simplest living form is the **cell**, the basic unit of life. Specialized cells are grouped into **tissues**, which, in turn, are combined to form **organs**; these organs form **systems**, which work together to maintain the body.

The systems are the

- integumentary system, the body's covering
- skeletal system, the framework of the body
- muscular system, which moves the bones and the skin of the face
- nervous system, the central control system that includes the organs of the sensory system
- endocrine system, which produces regulatory hormones
- cardiovascular system, consisting of the heart and blood vessels, acting to transport vital substances
- lymphatic system, which includes vessels that return tissue fluids to blood and organs that house immune cells
- respiratory system, which adds oxygen to the blood and removes carbon dioxide
- digestive system, which converts raw food materials into products usable by cells
- urinary system, which removes wastes and excess water
- reproductive system, by which new individuals of the species are produced

All the cellular reactions that sustain life together make up **metabolism**, which can be divided into **catabolism** and **anabolism**. In catabolism, complex substances are broken down into simpler molecules. When the nutrients from food are broken down by catabolism, energy is released. This energy is stored in the compound **ATP** (adenosine triphosphate) for use by the cells. In anabolism, simple compounds are built into substances needed for cell activities.

All the systems work together to maintain a state of balance or **homeostasis**. The main mechanism for maintaining homeostasis is **negative feedback**, by which the state of the body is the signal to keep conditions within set limits.

The human body is composed of large amounts of fluid, the amount and composition of which must be constantly regulated. The **extracellular fluid** consists of the fluid that surrounds the cells as well as the fluid circulating in blood and lymph. The fluid within cells is the **intracellular fluid**.

Study of the body requires knowledge of directional terms to locate parts and to relate various parts to each other. Planes of division represent different directions in which cuts can be made through the body. Separation of the body into areas and regions, together with the use of the special terminology for directions and locations, makes it possible to describe an area within the human body with great accuracy.

The large internal spaces of the body are cavities in which various organs are located. The **dorsal cavity** is subdivided into the **cranial cavity** and the **spinal cavity (canal)**. The **ventral cavity** is subdivided into the **thoracic** and **abdominopelvic cavities**. Imaginary lines are used to divide the abdomen into regions for study and diagnosis.

Addressing the Learning Outcomes

1. DEFINE THE TERMS *ANATOMY* AND *PHYSIOLOGY*.

EXERCISE 1-1

Write a definition of each term in the spaces below.

1. Anatomy _____

_____

2. Physiology _____

_____

2. DESCRIBE THE ORGANIZATION OF THE BODY FROM CHEMICALS TO THE WHOLE ORGANISM.

EXERCISE 1-2: Levels of Organization (Text Fig. 1-1)

1. Write the name or names of each labeled part on the numbered lines in different colors.
2. Color the different structures on the diagram with the corresponding color. For instance, if you wrote "cell" in blue, color the cell blue.

1. _____

2. _____

3. _____

4. _____

5. _____

6. _____

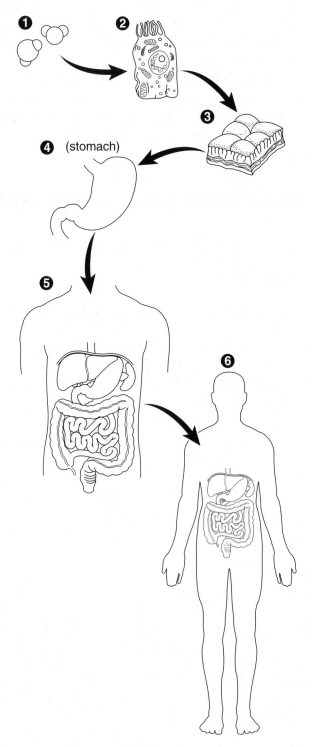

3. LIST 11 BODY SYSTEMS AND GIVE THE GENERAL FUNCTION OF EACH.

EXERCISE 1-3

Write the appropriate term in each blank from the list below.

nervous system	integumentary system	cardiovascular system
respiratory system	skeletal system	urinary system
endocrine system	lymphatic system	digestive system

1. The system that processes sensory information   _____

2. The system that delivers nutrients to body tissues   _____

3. The system that breaks down and absorbs food   _____

4. The system that includes the fingernails   _____

5. The system that includes the bladder   _____

6. The system that includes the joints   _____

7. The system that delivers oxygen to the blood   _____

8. The system that includes the tonsils   _____

4. DEFINE *METABOLISM* AND NAME THE TWO TYPES OF METABOLIC REACTIONS.

EXERCISE 1-4

Fill in the blanks in the paragraph below using the following terms: ATP, metabolism, catabolism, and anabolism.

The term _____ (1) refers to all life-sustaining reactions that occur within the body. The reactions involved in _____ (2) assemble simple components into more complex ones. The reactions of _____ (3) break down substances into simpler components, generating energy in the form of _____ (4). This energy can be used to fuel cell activities.

5. DEFINE AND GIVE EXAMPLES OF HOMEOSTASIS.

See Exercises 1-5 and 1-6.

6. EXPLAIN HOW NEGATIVE FEEDBACK MAINTAINS HOMEOSTASIS.

EXERCISE 1-5

Fill in the blanks in the paragraph below using the following terms: activates, shuts off, negative feedback, corrects, homeostasis.

The maintenance of a constant internal body state, known as (1) _____, is critical for health. Different body parameters, such as body temperature and blood glucose concentration, are kept constant using (2)_____ _____. For example, when the room temperature decreases, the thermostat (3) _____ the furnace to increase heat production. The resulting increase in room temperature (4) _____ the initial stimulus, and the thermostat (5)_____ the furnace.

EXERCISE 1-6

Homeostasis involves the regulation of body fluid volume and composition. Fill in the blank after each statement—does it apply to extracellular fluid (EC) or intracellular fluid (IC)?

1. Includes lymph and blood _____

2. Refers to fluids inside cells _____

3. Includes fluid between cells _____

7. LIST AND DEFINE THE MAIN DIRECTIONAL TERMS FOR THE BODY.

EXERCISE 1-7: Directional Terms (Text Fig. 1-6)

1. Write the name of each directional term on the numbered lines in different colors.
2. Color the arrow corresponding to each directional term with appropriate color.

1. _____

2. _____

3. _____

4. _____

5. _____

6. _____

7. _____

8. _____

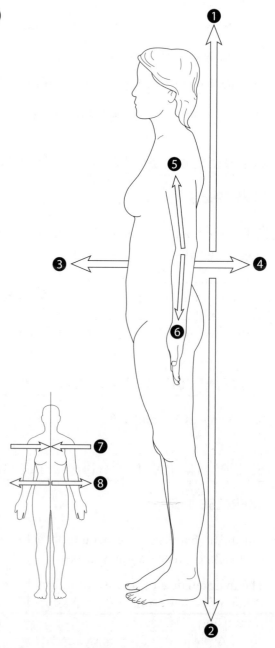

EXERCISE 1-8

Write the appropriate term in each blank from the list below.

posterior   anterior   medial   distal

proximal   lateral   horizontal

1. A term that indicates a location toward the front   _____

2. A term that means farther from the origin of a part   _____

3. A directional term that means away from the midline
   (toward the side)   _____

4. A term that describes the position of the ankle in relation
   to the toes   _____

5. A term that describes the position of the shoulder blades in
   relation to the collar bones   _____

8. LIST AND DEFINE THE THREE PLANES OF DIVISION OF THE BODY.

EXERCISE 1-9: Planes of Division (Text Fig. 1-7)

1. Write the names of the three planes of division on the correct numbered lines in different colors.
2. Color each plane in the illustration with its corresponding color.

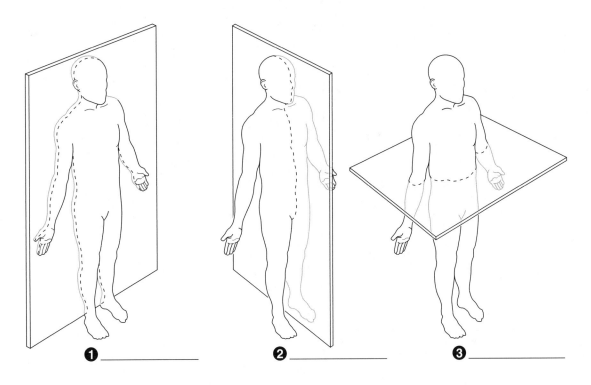

❶ _____   ❷ _____   ❸ _____

9. NAME THE SUBDIVISIONS OF THE DORSAL AND VENTRAL CAVITIES.

EXERCISE 1-10: Lateral View of Body Cavities (Text Fig. 1-10)

1. Write the names of the different body cavities and other structures in the appropriate spaces in different colors. Try to choose related colors for the dorsal cavity subdivisions and for the ventral cavity subdivisions.
2. Color parts 2, 3, and 6 to 9 with the corresponding color.

1. 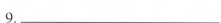_____

2. _____

3. _____

4. _____

5. _____

6. _____

7. _____

8. _____

9. _____

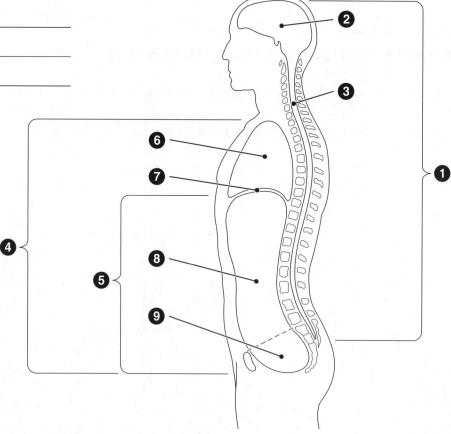

10. NAME AND LOCATE THE SUBDIVISIONS OF THE ABDOMEN.

EXERCISE 1-11: Regions of the Abdomen (Text Fig. 1-12)

1. Write the names of the nine regions of the abdomen on the appropriate numbered lines in different colors.
2. Color the corresponding region with the appropriate color.

1. _____

2. _____

3. _____

4. _____

5. _____

6. _____

7. _____

8. _____

9. _____

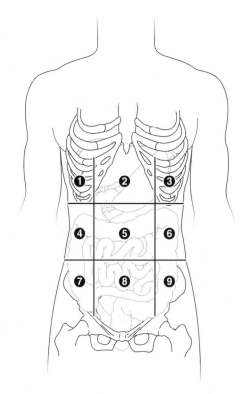

EXERCISE 1-12: Quadrants of the Abdomen (Text Fig. 1-13)

1. Write the names of the four quadrants of the abdomen on the appropriate numbered lines in different colors.
2. Color the corresponding quadrant in the appropriate color.

1. _____

2. _____

3. _____

4. _____

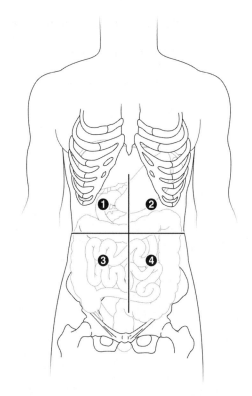

11. CITE SOME ANTERIOR AND POSTERIOR BODY REGIONS ALONG WITH THEIR COMMON NAMES.

EXERCISE 1-13

Complete the following table by writing in the missing terms.

Common Name	Anatomic Adjective
Thigh	
	Antecubital
	Inguinal
Arm	
Forearm	
	Axillary
	Tarsal
Shoulder blade	
	Acromial

12. FIND EXAMPLES OF ANATOMIC AND PHYSIOLOGIC TERMS IN A CASE STUDY.

EXERCISE 1-14

Read through the case study at the beginning of the chapter and the case study discussion at the end of the chapter. Find an example of each type of medical term listed below and write it in the blank.

a. A term describing one of four abdominal regions   _____

b. A term describing a particular region of the upper limb   _____

c. A term describing a body cavity   _____

d. A term describing one of nine abdominal regions   _____

e. A directional term   _____

13. SHOW HOW WORD PARTS ARE USED TO BUILD WORDS RELATED TO THE BODY'S ORGANIZATION.

EXERCISE 1-15

Complete the following table by writing the correct word part or meaning in the space provided. Write a word that contains each word part in the "Example" column.

Word Part	Meaning	Example
1. -tomy	_____	_____
2. -stasis	_____	_____
3. _____	nature, physical	_____
4. home/o	_____	_____
5. _____	apart, away from	_____
6. _____	down	_____
7. _____	upward	_____
8. -logy	_____	_____

Making the Connections

The following concept map deals with the body's cavities and their divisions. Complete the concept map by filling in the blanks with the appropriate word or term for the cavity, division, subdivision, or region.

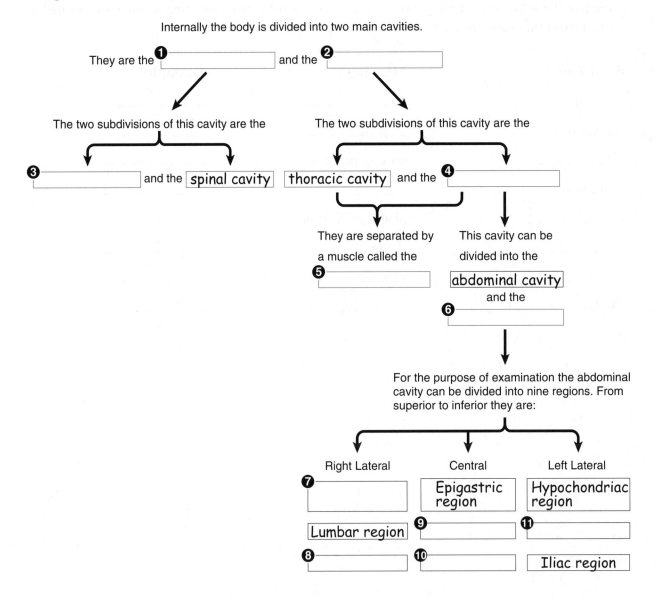

Testing Your Knowledge

BUILDING UNDERSTANDING

I. MULTIPLE CHOICE

Select the best answer and write the letter of your choice in the blank.

1. Which of these phrases describes a wart on the fingertip?   1._____
    a. phalangeal wart
    b. pedal wart
    c. tarsal wart
    d. axillary wart
2. Which two body cavities are separated by the diaphragm?   2. _____
    a. cranial and the spinal cavities
    b. dorsal and ventral cavities
    c. thoracic and abdominal cavities
    d. abdominal and pelvic cavities
3. What term describes the breakdown of complex molecules into more simple ones?   3. _____
    a. anabolism
    b. synthesis
    c. negative feedback
    d. catabolism
4. Blood plasma is an example of which type of fluid?   4. _____
    a. extracellular
    b. intracellular
    c. superior
    d. extraneous
5. Which body system consists of the skin and accessory organs?   5. _____
    a. circulatory system
    b. nervous system
    c. integumentary system
    d. digestive system
6. Which of these terms describes the right superior region of the abdomen?   6. _____
    a. right lumbar region
    b. right hypochondriac region
    c. right iliac region
    d. right inguinal region
7. Which of these terms describes the study of normal body structure?   7. _____
    a. physiology
    b. pathology
    c. anatomy
    d. homeostasis
8. Which of these sections is created when you cut a banana right down the middle, making two identical halves?   8. _____
    a. longitudinal section
    b. horizontal section
    c. cross section
    d. coronal section

II. COMPLETION EXERCISE

➤ Group A: General Terminology

Write the word or phrase that correctly completes each sentence.

1. In the anatomic position, the body is upright and palms are facing _____.

2. Fluid inside cells is called _____.

3. Catabolism releases energy in the form of _____.

4. Homeostasis is maintained by a form of feedback known as _____.

5. The sum of all catabolic and anabolic reactions in the body is called _____.

6. The abbreviation ATP stands for _____.

➤ Group B: Body Cavities, Directional Terms, and Planes Of Division

1. The term that means nearer to the point of origin is _____.

2. The term that means farther from the body's midline is _____.

3. The abdomen may be divided into four regions, each of which is called a(n) _____.

4. The cavity that houses the brain is the _____.

5. The plane that divides the body into left and right parts is the _____.

6. The ventral body cavity that contains the stomach, most of the intestine, the liver, and the spleen is the _____.

7. The abdomen may be subdivided into nine regions, including three along the midline. The region closest to the sternum (breastbone) is the _____.

8. The space between the lungs is called the _____.

9. The diaphragm separates the thoracic cavity from the _____.

➤ Group C: Body Regions

Write the anatomic adjective that corresponds to each body region.

1. Buttock _____

2. Wrist _____

3. Back of knee _____

4. Hip _____

5. Forearm _____

UNDERSTANDING CONCEPTS

I. TRUE/FALSE

For each question, write T for true or F for false in the blank to the left of each number. If a statement is false, correct it by replacing the <u>underlined</u> term and write the correct statement in the blank below the question.

_____ 1. Proteins are broken down into their component parts by the process of <u>catabolism</u>.

_____

_____ 2. The calcaneal tendon is most likely found in the <u>heel</u>.

_____

_____ 3. The spinal cavity is <u>superior</u> to the cranial cavity.

_____

_____ 4. Your umbilicus is <u>lateral</u> to the left lumbar region.

_____

_____ 5. The right hypochondriac region is found in the <u>right lower quadrant</u>.

_____

II. PRACTICAL APPLICATIONS

Study each discussion. Then write the appropriate word or phrase in the space provided.

➤ **Group A: Directional Terms**

1. The gallbladder is located just above the colon. The directional term that describes the position of the gallbladder with regard to the colon is _____.

2. The stomach is closer to the midline than the kidneys. The directional term that describes the kidneys with regard to the stomach is _____.

3. The entrance to the stomach is nearest the point of origin or beginning of the stomach, so this part is said to be _____.

4. The knee is located closer to the hip (the point of origin for the lower limb) than is the ankle. The term that describes the position of the ankle with regard to the knee is _____.

5. A child suffered from a burn extending from the umbilicus to the sternum. The term that describes the umbilical region in relation to the hypogastric region is _____.

6. The sternum is closer to the front of the body than the vertebrae. The term that describes the vertebrae with regard to the sternum is _____.

7. The head of the pancreas is nearer the midsagittal plane than is its tail portion, so the head part is more _____.

➤ Group B: Body Cavities and Body Regions

Study the following cases and answer the questions based on the nine divisions of the abdomen and the anatomic terms for body regions.

1. Mr. A bruised his ribs in a dirt buggy accident. He experienced tenderness in the upper left side of his abdomen. In which of the nine abdominal regions are the injured ribs located?
   _____

2. Ms. D had a history of gallstones. One of her symptoms was referred pain between the shoulder blades. The adjective describing the shoulder blade is _____.

3. The operation to remove these stones involved the upper right part of the abdominal cavity. Which abdominal division is this? _____

4. Ms. C is 8 weeks pregnant. Her uterus is still confined to the most inferior division of the abdomen. This cavity is called the _____.

5. Ms. C is experiencing heartburn as a result of her pregnancy. The discomfort is found just below the breastbone, in the _____.

6. When she went into labor, she experienced significant pain in the small of her back. What is the anatomical adjective describing this region? _____

7. Following the birth of her child, Ms. C opted for a tubal ligation. The doctor threaded a fiber-optic device through a small incision in her navel as part of the surgery. Ms. C will now have a very small incision in which of the nine abdominal regions? _____

➤ Group C: Body Systems

The triage nurse in the Emergency Room was showing a group of students how she assessed patients with disorders in different body systems. Study each situation, and answer the following questions based on your knowledge of the 11 body systems.

1. One person was complaining of dizziness and blurred vision. Vision is controlled by the _____.

2. One person had been injured in a snowboarding accident, spraining his wrist joint. The wrist joint is part of the _____.

3. A woman had attempted a particularly onerous yoga pose, and felt a sharp pain in her left thigh. Now she was limping. The nurse suspected a tear to structures belonging to the _____.

4. An extremely tall individual entered the clinic, complaining of a headache. The nurse suspected that he had excess production of a particular hormone. The specialized glands that synthesize hormones make up the _____.

5. A middle-aged woman was brought in unable to move the right side of her body. The nurse felt that a blood clot in a blood vessel of the brain was producing the symptoms. Blood vessels are part of the _____.

6. A man complaining of pain in the abdomen and vomiting blood was brought in by his family. A problem was suspected in the system responsible for taking in food and converting it to usable products. This system is the _____.

7. Each client was assessed for changes in the color of the outer covering of the body. The outer covering is called the skin, which is part of the _____.

8. A young woman was experiencing pain in her pelvic region. The doctor suspected a problem with her ovaries. The ovaries are part of the _____.

9. An older man was experiencing difficulty with urination. The production of urine is the function of the _____.

III. SHORT ESSAYS

1. Compare and contrast the terms *anabolism* and *catabolism*. List one similarity and one difference.

   _____

   _____

   _____

   _____

   _____

2. What is homeostasis, and how does negative feedback help to maintain it?

   _____

   _____

   _____

   _____

3. Explain why specialized terms are needed to indicate different positions, regions, and directions within the body. Provide a concrete example.

   _____

   _____

   _____

   _____

   _____

CONCEPTUAL THINKING

1. In the lines below, rewrite this description replacing all underlined words with precise anatomic terms.

   "A 40-year-old man was brought into the ER suffering from multiple wounds. One laceration was in the <u>shoulder blade</u> region, just <u>above</u> a mole. The second was in his <u>calf</u> region, <u>farther from the midline than</u> a scar from a previous injury. Finally, he had multiple small cuts extending from the <u>abdominal region just below his sternum</u> to the region <u>overlying his left hip bone</u>."

   _____

   _____

   _____

   _____

   _____

   _____

2. Look back at the case study at the beginning of the chapter, and answer the following questions.
   a. What was the main challenge to Mike's homeostasis (hint: the numbers involved are 80 and 40)?
   b. How did his heart try to compensate for this challenge?
   c. Which body system contains the heart?
   d. Find two medical interventions *performed by the paramedics* that helped Mike deal with his homeostatic challenge.

   a. _____

   _____

   b. _____

   _____

   c. _____

   _____

   d. _____

   _____

3. A disease at the chemical level can have an effect on the whole body. That is, a change in a chemical affects a cell, which alters the functioning of a tissue, which disrupts an organ, which disrupts a system, which results in body dysfunction. Illustrate this concept by rewriting the following description in your own words using the different levels of organization in order of complexity: chemical, cell, tissue, organ, system, and body (hint: blood is a tissue). Your answer should address the following issues: (a) Which of the bold terms applies to each level of organization? (b) Which level of organization is not explicitly stated in the question?

Mr. S. experiences pain throughout his **body**. The movement of **blood** through his **blood vessels** is impaired. His **blood cells** are misshapen. A chemical found in red blood cells called **hemoglobin** is abnormal.

_____

_____

_____

_____

_____

_____

Expanding Your Horizons

As a student of anatomy and physiology, you have joined a community of scholars stretching back into prehistory. The history of biological thought is a fascinating one, full of murder and intrigue. We think that scientific knowledge is entirely objective. However, as the books below will show, theories of anatomy, physiology, and disease depend upon societal factors such as economic class, religion, and gender issues.

- Endersby J. A Guinea Pig's History of Biology. Cambridge, MA. Harvard University Press, 2009.
- History of Anatomy. Available at: http://www.historyworld.net/wrldhis/PlainTextHistories.asp?groupid=44&HistoryID=aa05&gtrack=pthc
- Luft EVD. History of Anatomy and Physiology: The Classical and Medieval Periods. Available at: http://www.bookrags.com/research/history-of-anatomy-and-physiology-t-wap/
- Magner LN. A History of the Life Sciences. Boca Raton, FL: CRC Press, 2003.

CHAPTER
2
Chemistry, Matter, and Life

Overview

Chemistry is the physical science that deals with the composition of matter. To appreciate the importance of chemistry in the field of health, it is necessary to know about elements, atoms, molecules, compounds, and mixtures. An **element** is a substance consisting of just one type of atom. Although exceedingly small particles, atoms possess a definite structure. The **nucleus** contains **protons** and **neutrons**, and the element's **atomic number** indicates the number of protons in its nucleus. The **electrons** surround the nucleus where they are arranged in specific orbits called **energy levels**.

If an atom does not have enough electrons to fill its outermost energy level, it will interact with other atoms, forming a **chemical bond**. The transfer of electrons from one atom to another results in an **ionic bond**. The participating atoms now have an uneven number of protons and electrons, so they have an electric charge and are called **ions**. Ions serve many important roles in the body. Ionically bonded substances tend to separate into their component ions in solution. Bonds that form when two atoms share electrons between them are called **covalent bonds**. Covalent bonds are usually very strong; they result in the formation of **molecules**. The atoms in the molecule may be alike (as in the oxygen molecule, O_2) or different (as in water, H_2O). A **compound** is any substance composed of more than one type of atom. So, oxygen (O_2) is a molecule but not a compound, but NaCl (which is formed by ionic bonds) is a compound but not a molecule. A combination of substances, each of which retains its separate properties, is a **mixture**. Mixtures include solutions, such as salt water, and suspensions.

Water is a vital substance composed of hydrogen and oxygen. It makes up more than half of the body and is needed as a solvent and a transport medium. Hydrogen, oxygen, carbon, and nitrogen are the elements that constitute about 96% of living matter, whereas calcium, sodium, potassium, phosphorus, sulfur, chlorine, and magnesium account for most of the remaining 4%.

Inorganic compounds include acids, bases, and salts. **Acids** are compounds that can donate hydrogen ions (H^+) when in solution. **Bases** can accept hydrogen ions and usually contain the hydroxide ion (OH^-). The **pH scale** is used to indicate the strength of an acid or base. **Salts** are formed when an acid reacts with a base. The components of a salt are always joined by ionic bonds.

Isotopes are forms of elements that vary in neutron number. Isotopes that give off radiation are said to be **radioactive**. Because they can penetrate tissues and can be traced in the body, they are useful in diagnosis. Radioactive substances also have the ability to destroy tissues and can be used in the treatment of many types of cancer.

Proteins, carbohydrates, and lipids are the organic compounds characteristic of living organisms. Each type of organic compound is built from characteristic building blocks. **Enzymes**, an important group of proteins, function as catalysts in metabolism. **Nucleotides** are a fourth type of organic compound. Important molecules built from nucleotides include DNA, RNA, and ATP.

Addressing the Learning Outcomes

1. DEFINE A CHEMICAL ELEMENT.

See Exercise 2-1.

2. DESCRIBE THE STRUCTURE OF AN ATOM.

EXERCISE 2-1

Write the appropriate term in each blank from the list below.

nucleus	proton	element	electron
neutron	atom	energy level	

1. A positively charged particle inside the atomic nucleus   _____

2. The smallest complete unit of matter   _____

3. An uncharged particle inside the atomic nucleus   _____

4. A substance composed of one type of atom   _____

5. The part of the atom containing protons and neutrons   _____

6. A negatively charged particle outside the atomic nucleus   _____

EXERCISE 2-2: Parts of the Atom, Molecule of Water (Text Figs. 2-1 and 2-5)

1. This figure illustrates two hydrogen atoms and one oxygen atom. Write the names of the parts of the atom (electron, proton, neutron) on the appropriate lines in different, darker colors.
2. Color the electrons, protons, and neutrons on the figure in the appropriate colors. You should find 10 electrons, 10 protons, and 8 neutrons in total.
3. Use two contrasting, light colors to shade the first energy level (4) and the second energy level (5).

1. _____
2. _____
3. _____
4. _____
5. _____

3. DIFFERENTIATE BETWEEN IONIC AND COVALENT BONDS.

See Exercise 2-3.

4. DEFINE AN ELECTROLYTE.

EXERCISE 2-3

Write the appropriate term in each blank from the list below.

cations   ionic   nonpolar covalent

electrolytes   anions   polar covalent

1. Negatively charged ions   _____

2. A bond formed by the equal sharing of electrons between two
   atoms   _____

3. Compounds that form ions when in solution   _____

4. Positively charged ions   _____

5. A bond formed by the transfer of electron(s) from one atom
   to another   _____

6. A bond formed by the unequal sharing of electrons between
   two atoms   _____

5. DIFFERENTIATE BETWEEN MOLECULES AND COMPOUNDS.

EXERCISE 2-4

Fill in the blank after each statement—does it apply to molecules (M), compounds (C), or both (B)?

1. Contain two or more atoms _____

2. Contain two identical atoms _____

3. Always contain two different atoms _____

4. Can consist of two identical covalently bonded atoms _____

5. Can consist of two different covalently bonded atoms _____

6. Can consist of two different ionically bonded atoms _____

6. DEFINE *MIXTURE*; LIST THE THREE TYPES OF MIXTURES, AND GIVE TWO EXAMPLES OF EACH.

EXERCISE 2-5

Write the appropriate term in each blank from the list below.

solution	suspension	solute
solvent	aqueous	mixture colloid

1. The substance in which another substance is dissolved _____

2. A substance that is dissolved in another substance _____

3. A mixture in which substances will settle out unless the mixture is shaken _____

4. Term used to describe a solution mostly formed of water _____

5. Cytosol and blood plasma are examples of this type of suspension _____

6. Any combination of two or more substances in which each constituent maintains its identity _____

7. EXPLAIN WHY WATER IS SO IMPORTANT IN METABOLISM.

EXERCISE 2-6

Which of the following properties are NOT true of water? There is one correct answer.

   a. All substances can dissolve in water.
   b. Water participates in chemical reactions.
   c. Water is a stable liquid at ordinary temperatures.
   d. Water carries substances to and from cells.

8. COMPARE ACIDS, BASES, AND SALTS.

See Exercise 2-7.

9. EXPLAIN HOW THE NUMBERS ON THE pH SCALE RELATE TO ACIDITY AND ALKALINITY.

See Exercise 2-7.

10. EXPLAIN WHY BUFFERS ARE IMPORTANT IN THE BODY.

EXERCISE 2-7

Fill in the blanks in the paragraph below using the following terms: pH scale, salt, acid, base, buffer, hydroxide, alkali, hydrogen, high, low.

Any substance that can donate a hydrogen ion to another substance is called a(n) (1)_____. Any substance that can accept a hydrogen ion is called a(n) (2) _____ or a(n) (3)_____. Many of these contain a(n) (4) _____ ion. A reaction between a hydrogen-accepting substance and a hydrogen-donating substance produces a(n) (5) _____. The (6)_____ measures the concentration of hydrogen ions in a solution. A solution with a large concentration of hydrogen ions will have a(n) (7) _____ pH; a solution with a large concentration of hydroxide ions will have a(n) (8) _____ pH. A substance that helps to maintain a stable hydrogen ion concentration in a solution is called a(n) (9) _____; these substances are critical for health.

11. DEFINE *RADIOACTIVITY* AND CITE SEVERAL EXAMPLES OF HOW RADIOACTIVE SUBSTANCES ARE USED IN MEDICINE.

EXERCISE 2-8

Which of the following statements about radioactivity are TRUE? There are four right answers.

a. All isotopes are radioactive.
b. Isotopes have the same atomic weight.
c. Isotopes have the same number of protons.
d. Isotopes have the same number of electrons.
e. Isotopes have the same number of neutrons.
f. Radioactive isotopes disintegrate easily.
g. Radioactive isotopes can be used for diagnosis and treatment.

12. NAME THE THREE MAIN TYPES OF ORGANIC COMPOUNDS AND THE BUILDING BLOCKS OF EACH.

EXERCISE 2-9

Write the appropriate term in each blank from the list below.

carbon	protein	amino acid	phospholipid	carbohydrate
monosaccharide	steroid	disaccharide	nitrogen	

1. A building block always containing nitrogen _____

2. The nutrient formed by amino acids _____

3. A lipid containing a ring of carbon atoms _____

4. A lipid that contains phosphorus in addition to carbon, hydrogen, and oxygen _____

5. A category of organic compounds that includes simple sugars and starches

_____

6. The element found in all organic compounds

_____

7. A building block for complex carbohydrates

_____

EXERCISE 2-10: Carbohydrates (Text Fig. 2-8)

1. Write the terms _disaccharide, monosaccharide,_ and _polysaccharide_ in the appropriate numbered boxes 1 to 3.
2. Write the terms _sucrose, glycogen,_ and _glucose_ in the appropriate numbered boxes 4 to 6 in different colors.
3. Color the glucose, sucrose, and glycogen molecules with the appropriate colors. To simplify your diagram, only use the glucose color to shade the glucose molecule in the monosaccharide.

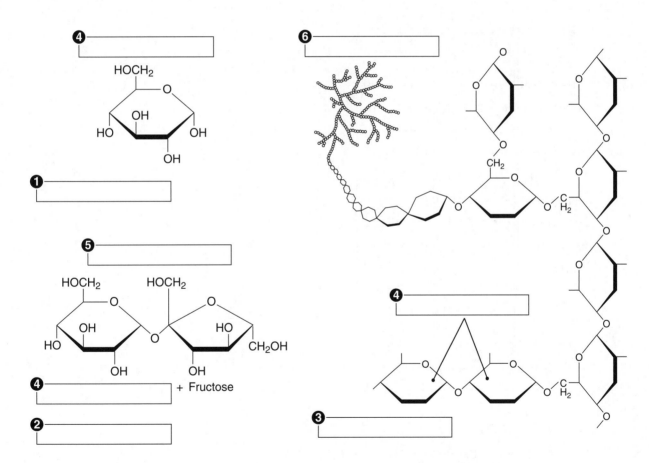

EXERCISE 2-11: Lipids (Text Fig. 2-9)

➤ **Instructions**

1. Write the terms *fatty acids* and *glycerol* on the appropriate lines in two different colors.
2. Find the boxes surrounding these two components on the diagram, and color them lightly in the appropriate colors.
3. Write the terms *cholesterol* and *triglyceride* in the boxes under the appropriate diagrams.

1. _____

2. _____

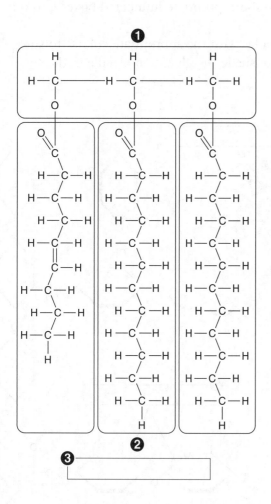

EXERCISE 2-12: Proteins (Text Fig. 2-10)

1. Write the terms *acid group* and *amino group* on the appropriate numbered lines in different colors.
2. Find the shapes surrounding these two components on the diagram, and color them lightly in the appropriate colors.
3. Place the following terms in the appropriate numbered boxes: amino acid, coiled, pleated, folded.

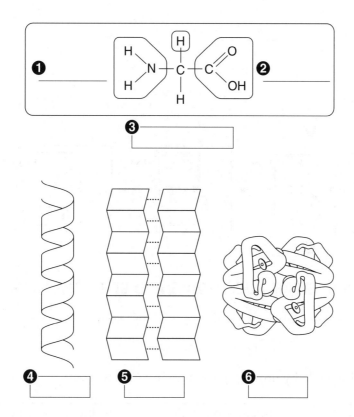

13. DEFINE *ENZYME* AND DESCRIBE HOW ENZYMES WORK.

EXERCISE 2-13: Enzyme Action (Text Fig. 2-11)

1. Write the terms *enzyme, substrate 1,* and *substrate 2* on the appropriate numbered lines in different colors (red and blue are recommended for the substrates).
2. Color the structures on the diagram with the appropriate color.
3. What color will result from the combination of your two substrate colors? Write "product" in this color on the appropriate line, and then color the product.

1. _____

2. _____

3. _____

4. _____

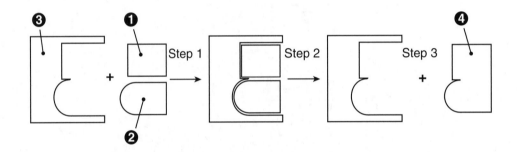

14. LIST THE COMPONENTS OF NUCLEOTIDES AND GIVE SOME EXAMPLES OF NUCLEOTIDES.

EXERCISE 2-14

Complete the following table by providing the missing information.

Building Blocks	Finished Product	Purpose of Finished Product or Example
	Triglyceride (simple fat)	Purpose:
2 monosaccharides		Example:
1 monosaccharide	Monosaccharide	Example:
Many monosaccharides		Examples: starch, glycogen
	Protein	Purpose:
One nucleotide containing three phosphate groups		Purpose:
	DNA or RNA	Purpose:

EXERCISE 2-15

Indicate whether each of the following components is part of an amino acid (A) or a nucleotide (N) by writing the appropriate letter in each blank.

1. Phosphate group _____

2. Amino group _____

3. Nitrogenous base _____

4. Sugar _____

5. Acid group _____

6. Side chain (R group) _____

15. USE THE CASE STUDY TO DISCUSS THE IMPORTANCE OF BODY FLUID QUANTITY AND COMPOSITION.

EXERCISE 2-16

Use the terms below to complete the paragraph. One term will not be used.

increased   **decreased**   **sodium**   **high blood pressure**   **low blood pressure**

Margaret Ringland presented many signs of dehydration. Without adequate water, her blood volume (1) _____, resulting in hypotension, or (2) _____. Her body tried to compensate, so it (3) _____ her heart rate. Without enough water, the concentration of (4) _____, abbreviated as Na, was elevated.

16. SHOW HOW WORD PARTS ARE USED TO BUILD WORDS RELATED TO CHEMISTRY, MATTER, AND LIFE.

EXERCISE 2-17

Complete the following table by writing the correct word part or meaning in the space provided. Write a word that contains each word part in the Example column.

Word Part	Meaning	Example
1. _____	fear	_____
2. _____	to like	_____
3. glyc/o	_____	_____
4. _____	different	_____
5. hydr/o	_____	_____
6. hom/o-	_____	_____
7. _____	many	_____
8. -ase	_____	_____
9. sacchar/o	_____	_____
10. _____	together	_____

Making the Connections

The following concept map deals with the three major types of nutrients. Complete the concept map by filling in the blanks with the appropriate word or term.

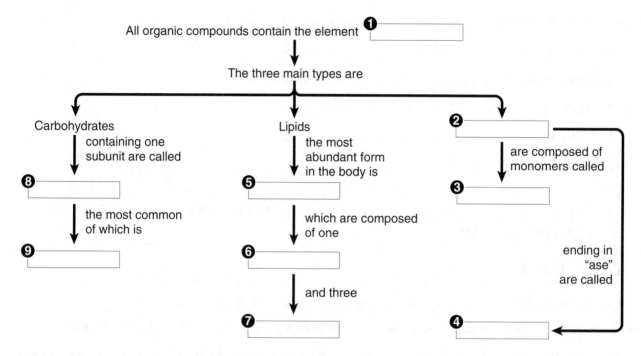

All organic compounds contain the element **❶** [   ]

The three main types are

Carbohydrates
  containing one subunit are called
  ❽ [   ]
  the most common of which is
  ❾ [   ]

Lipids
  the most abundant form in the body is
  ❺ [   ]
  which are composed of one
  ❻ [   ]
  and three
  ❼ [   ]

❷ [   ]
  are composed of monomers called
  ❸ [   ]

  ending in "ase" are called
  ❹ [   ]

Optional Exercise: Construct your own concept map using the following terms: atom, nucleus, electron, proton, neutron, energy level, covalent bond, ionic bond.

Testing Your Knowledge

BUILDING UNDERSTANDING

I. MULTIPLE CHOICE

Select the best answer and write the letter of your choice in the blank.

1. Which of these terms best describes a solution with a pH of 3?   1. _____
   a. basic
   b. acidic
   c. neutral
   d. hydrophobic

2. Which of these terms describes the smallest particle of an element that has all the properties of that element?   2. _____
   a. proton
   b. neutron
   c. electron
   d. atom

3. Which of these terms describes the particle that results when
an electron is added to an atom?   3. _____
    a. proton
    b. anion
    c. cation
    d. electrolyte

4. Which of these phrases best describes the different orbits
that electrons can occupy?   4. _____
    a. energy levels
    b. ellipses
    c. pathways
    d. isotopes

5. What sort of macromolecule is ATP?   5. _____
    a. protein
    b. amino acid
    c. nucleotide
    d. lipid

6. Which of these is a building block for lipids?   6. _____
    a. amino acids
    b. free fatty acids
    c. nucleotides
    d. monosaccharides

7. Which of these phrases best describes covalent bonds?   7. _____
    a. usually formed between two ions
    b. can be classified as polar or nonpolar
    c. never used in organic molecules
    d. usually very unstable

8. What type of solution results when salt completely dissolves
in water?   8. _____
    a. colloid
    b. suspension
    c. aqueous solution
    d. isotope

9. What is an alternate term for a complex carbohydrate?   9. _____
    a. polysaccharide
    b. lipid
    c. inorganic molecule
    d. isotope

II. COMPLETION EXERCISE

Write the word or phrase that correctly completes each sentence.

1. All organic compounds contain the element _____.

2. The number of electrons lost or gained by an atom in a chemical reaction is called its _____.

3. Water can dissolve many different things. For this reason, it is called the _____.

4. The atoms in hydrogen gas (H_2) and in water (H_2O) are joined together by covalent bonds. Both of these substances are thus composed of _____.

5. An isotope that disintegrates, giving off rays of atomic particles, is said to be _____.

6. A mixture that is not a solution but does not separate because the particles in the mixture are so small is a(n) _____.

7. Many essential body activities depend on certain compounds that form ions when in solution. Such compounds are called _____.

8. The name given to a chemical system that prevents changes in hydrogen ion concentration is _____.

9. The study of the composition and properties of matter is called _____.

10. Metabolic reactions require organic catalysts called _____.

UNDERSTANDING CONCEPTS

I. TRUE/FALSE

For each question, write T for true or F for false in the blank to the left of each number. If a statement is false, correct it by replacing the underlined term and write the correct statement in the blank below the question.

_____ 1. Sodium chloride (NaCl) is an example of an underlined element.

_____

_____ 2. If a neutral atom has 12 protons, it will have 11 electrons.

_____

_____ 3. An atom with an atomic number of 22 will have 22 protons.

_____

_____ 4. Sugar dissolves easily in water. Sugar is thus an example of a <u>hydrophobic</u> substance.

_____

_____ 5. When table salt is dissolved in water, the sodium ion donates one electron to the chloride ion. The chloride ion has 17 protons, so it will have <u>16</u> electrons.

_____

_____ 6. You put some soil in water and shake well. After 10 minutes, you note that some of the dirt has settled to the bottom of the jar. With respect to the dirt at the bottom of the jar, your mixture is a <u>colloid</u>.

_____

_____ 7. A pH of 7.0 is <u>basic</u>.

_____

_____ 8. Oxygen gas is composed of two oxygen atoms bonded by the sharing of electrons. Oxygen gas is formed by <u>polar covalent bonds</u>.

_____

_____ 9. Glycogen, a <u>polysaccharide,</u> is composed of many glucose molecules.

_____

_____ 10. Nucleotides contain three building blocks: a nitrogenous base, a sugar, and an <u>amino acid</u>.

_____

II. PRACTICAL APPLICATIONS

Study each discussion. Then write the appropriate word or phrase in the space provided. The following medical tests are based on principles of chemistry and physics.

1. Young Ms. M was experiencing intense thirst and was urinating more than usual. Her doctor suspected that she might have diabetes mellitus. This diagnosis was confirmed by finding of ketones in her urine. Ketones result from the partial breakdown of fatty acids. Fatty acids, along with glycerol, form simple fats, which are also known as _____.

2. The pH of Ms. M's urine was lower than normal, reflecting the presence of the ketones. Ketones donate hydrogen ions to other molecules, so they can be described as _____.

3. The presence of ketones changed the pH of Ms. M's urine. The pH of her urine was _____ than normal.

4. Ms. M's urine also contained large amounts of glucose. Each glucose molecule consists of a single sugar unit, so glucose is an example of a(n) _____.

5. Because of Ms. M's excessive urination, she was suffering from dehydration. Her intense thirst reflects a shortage of the most abundant compound in the body, which is

   _____.

6. Mr. Q has been experiencing diarrhea, intestinal gas, and bloating whenever he drinks milk. He was diagnosed with a deficiency in an enzyme called lactase, which digests the sugar in milk. Enzymes, like all proteins, are composed of building blocks called

   _____.

7. Daredevil Mr. L was riding his skateboard on a high wall when he fell. He had pain and swelling in his right wrist. His examination included a procedure in which rays penetrate body tissues to produce an image on a photographic plate. The rays used for this purpose are called _____.

8. Ms. F. was given an intravenous solution, containing sodium, potassium, and chloride ions. These elements come from salts that separate into ions in solution and are referred to as

   _____.

III. SHORT ESSAYS

1. Describe the structure of a protein. Make sure you include the following terms in your answer: pleated sheet, helix, protein, peptide bond, amino acid.

   _____

   _____

   _____

   _____

   _____

2. What is the difference between a solvent and a solute? Name the solvent and the solute in salt water.

   _____

   _____

   _____

   _____

   _____

3. Why is the shape of an enzyme important in its function?

   _____

   _____

   _____

   _____

   _____

4. Compare and contrast colloids and suspensions. Name at least one similarity and one difference.

_____

_____

_____

_____

_____

CONCEPTUAL THINKING

1. Using the periodic table of the elements in Appendix 1, answer the following questions:
   a. How many protons does calcium (Ca) have? _____
   b. How many electrons does nitrogen (N) have? _____
   c. Phosphorus (P) exists as many isotopes. One isotope is called P^{32}, based on its atomic weight. The atomic weight can be calculated by adding up the number of protons and the number of neutrons. How many neutrons does P^{32} have? _____
   d. How many electrons does the magnesium ion Mg^{2+} have? (The 2+ indicates that the magnesium atom has lost two electrons). _____

2. There is much more variety in proteins than in complex carbohydrates. Explain why.

_____

_____

_____

3. Read each of the following descriptions. State whether each description pertains to molecules (M), compounds (C), and/or electrolytes (E) by writing the correct letter(s) in the blank. More than one term may apply to each description.
   a. Hydrochloric acid (HCl) dissociates completely into an H^+ ion and a Cl^- ion when dissolved in water. _____
   b. Methane (CH_4) contains one atom of carbon that forms nonpolar covalent bonds with four different hydrogen atoms. _____
   c. Nitrous oxide (N_2O) is also known as laughing gas. It consists of one nitrogen atom that forms polar covalent bonds with two different oxygen atoms. _____
   d. If nitrogen gas (N_2) is cooled to a very low temperature, it forms a liquid that can freeze a grape solid in 2 seconds. _____

Expanding Your Horizons

1. You may have read the term *antioxidant* in newspaper articles or on the Web. But what is an antioxidant, and why do we want them? An understanding of atomic structure is required to answer this question. Radiation or chemical reactions can cause molecules to pick up or lose an electron, resulting in an unpaired electron. Molecules with unpaired electrons are called **free radicals.** For instance, an oxygen molecule can gain an electron, resulting in superoxide (O_2^-). Most free radicals produced in humans contain oxygen, so they are called **reactive oxygen species (ROS).** Unpaired electrons are very unstable; thus, free radicals steal electrons from other substances, converting them into free radicals. This chain reaction disrupts normal cell metabolism and can result in cancer and other diseases. Antioxidants, including vitamin C, give up electrons without converting into free radicals, thereby stopping the chain reaction. The references listed below will tell you more about free radicals and antioxidants.

   - Brown K. A radical proposal. Sci Am Presents 2000;11:38–43.
   - National Cancer Institute. Available at: http://www.cancer.gov/cancertopics/factsheet/prevention/antioxidants
   - Waris G, Ahsan H. Reactive oxygen species: role in the development of cancer and various chronic conditions. J Carcinog 2006;5:14. Available at: http://www.ncbi.nlm.nih.gov/pmc/articles/PMC1479806/

2. Proteins are the "nanomachines of life," accomplishing all of the functions needed to keep us alive. For decades scientists have tried to create synthetic proteins of a particular shape to serve a particular function, such as blocking the sites the cholera toxin uses to create diarrhea. But, despite extensive efforts, scientists still have no way of predicting the final shape of a protein based on its amino acid sequence. Without this information, it is difficult to develop proteins to serve a particular purpose. Scientists are turning to synthetic building blocks called bis-amino acids that assume more predictable conformations when they are joined together. You can read more about the prospects of these "molecular lego blocks" in the reference below.

   - Schafmeister CE. Molecular Lego. *Scientific American* 2007;296:76–82B.

CHAPTER

3

Cells and Their Functions

Overview

The **cell** is the basic unit of life; all life activities result from the activities of cells. The study of cells began with the invention of the light microscope and has continued with the development of electron microscopes. Cell functions are carried out by specialized structures within the cell called **organelles**. These include the nucleus, ribosomes, mitochondria, Golgi apparatus, endoplasmic reticulum (ER), lysosomes, peroxisomes, and centrioles. Two specialized organelles, cilia and flagella, function in cell locomotion and the movement of materials across the cell surface.

The **plasma (cell) membrane** is important in regulating what enters and leaves the cell. Lipid-soluble substances can pass through the membrane by **simple diffusion**, which is simply the movement of molecules from an area where they are in higher concentration to an area where they are in lower concentration. This direction of movement is described as *down the concentration gradient*. Water-soluble substances require specialized proteins to *facilitate* their passage through the plasma membrane, so they move down their concentration gradients by **facilitated diffusion.**

Water also crosses the plasma membrane, down its concentration gradient, with the aid of membrane proteins called *aquaporins*. This process is called **osmosis**. Since the water and solute concentrations are inversely related, water moves from the area of *low* solute concentration to the region with a *high* solute concentration. Osmosis changes cell volume, so it must be prevented by keeping cells in solutions that have the same overall solute concentration as the cytosol. If the cell is placed in a solution of higher concentration, a **hypertonic solution**, it will shrink; in a solution of lower concentration, a **hypotonic solution**, it will swell and may burst.

Diffusion and osmosis use the energy of moving particles to drive movement. A different form of passive transport, **filtration**, uses pressure gradients to move substances from an area of high pressure to one of lower pressure.

The plasma membrane can also selectively move substances against the concentration gradient (from low concentration to high) by **active transport**, a process that requires energy (ATP) and transporters. Energy is also used to move large particles and droplets of fluid across the plasma membrane by the processes of **endocytosis** and **exocytosis**. Concentration gradients are not relevant to these vesicle-mediated processes.

An important cell function is the manufacture of proteins, including enzymes (organic catalysts). Protein manufacture is carried out by the ribosomes in the cytoplasm according to information coded in the deoxyribonucleic acid (DNA) of the nucleus. Specialized molecules of RNA, called messenger RNA, play a key role in the process by carrying copies of the information in DNA to the ribosomes. DNA also is involved in the process of cell division or mitosis. Before cell division can occur, the DNA must double itself by the process of DNA replication, so each daughter cell produced by mitosis will have exactly the same kind and amount of DNA as the parent cell.

Addressing the Learning Outcomes

1. LIST THREE TYPES OF MICROSCOPES USED TO STUDY CELLS.

EXERCISE 3-1

Write the appropriate term in each blank from the list below.

compound light microscope   transmission electron microscope

scanning electron microscope   micrometer   centimeter

1. 1/1,000 of a millimeter   _____

2. Microscope that provides a three-dimensional view of an object _____

3. The most common microscope, which magnifies an object up to 1,000 times _____

4. A microscope that magnifies an object up to one million times _____

2. DESCRIBE THE COMPOSITION AND FUNCTIONS OF THE PLASMA MEMBRANE.

EXERCISE 3-2: Structure of the Plasma Membrane (Text Fig. 3-3)

1. Write the name of each labeled membrane component on the numbered lines in different colors. Choose a light color for component number 3.
2. Color the different structures on the diagram with the corresponding color (except for structures 6 to 8). Color every example of components 1 through 5, not just those indicated by the leader lines. For instance, component 1 is found in three locations.

1. _____

2. _____

3. _____

4. _____

5. _____

6. _____

7. _____

8. _____

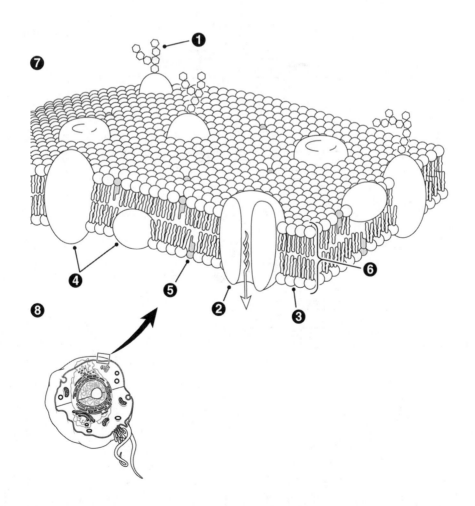

EXERCISE 3-3: Membrane Proteins (Table 3-1)

1. Write the appropriate membrane protein function in boxes 1 to 6 in different colors.
2. Color the protein in each diagram the appropriate color.

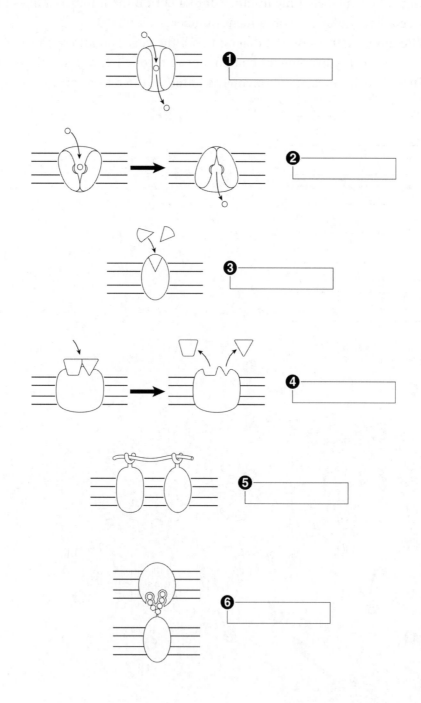

3. DESCRIBE THE CYTOPLASM OF THE CELL, INCLUDING THE NAME AND FUNCTION OF THE MAIN ORGANELLES.

EXERCISE 3-4: Typical Animal Cell Showing the Main Organelles (Text Fig. 3-2)

1. Write the name of each labeled part on the numbered lines in different colors. Make sure you use light colors for structures 1 and 7.
2. Color the different structures on the diagram with the corresponding color.

*Note: Parts 12 and 15 have the same appearance in this diagram; write the name of one of the possible options in blank 12 and the other in blank 15.

1. _____

2. _____

3. _____

4. _____

5. _____

6. _____

7. _____

8. _____

9. _____

10. _____

11. _____

12. _____

13. _____

14. _____

15. _____

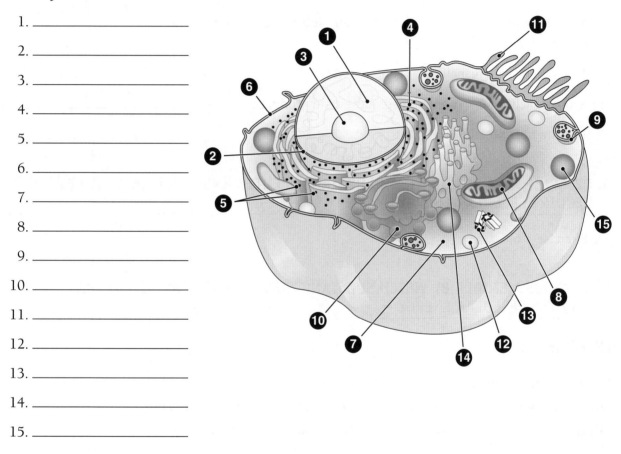

EXERCISE 3-5

Write the appropriate term in each blank from the list below.

lysosome	nucleolus	cilia	ribosome
mitochondrion	nucleus	Golgi apparatus	vesicle

1. A structure that assembles ribosomes _____

2. A structure that assembles amino acids into proteins _____

3. A set of membranes involved in packaging proteins for export _____

4. A small saclike structure used to transport substances within the cell _____

5. A membranous organelle that generates ATP _____

6. A small saclike structure that degrades waste products _____

7. The site of DNA storage _____

4. DESCRIBE METHODS BY WHICH SUBSTANCES ENTER AND LEAVE CELLS THAT DO NOT REQUIRE CELLULAR ENERGY

See Exercise 3-6.

5. DESCRIBE METHODS BY WHICH SUBSTANCES ENTER AND LEAVE CELLS THAT REQUIRE CELLULAR ENERGY

EXERCISE 3-6

Write the appropriate term in each blank from the list below.

facilitated diffusion	exocytosis	endocytosis	active transport
diffusion	osmosis	filtration	pinocytosis

1. The process that utilizes a carrier to move materials across the plasma membrane against the concentration gradient using ATP _____

2. The use of hydrostatic force to move fluids through a membrane _____

3. The process that utilizes a carrier to move materials across the plasma membrane in the direction of theconcentration gradient _____

4. A special form of diffusion that applies only to water _____

5. The spread of molecules throughout an area   _____

6. The process by which a cell takes in large particles   _____

7. The process by which materials are expelled from the cell using vesicles   _____

8. Small fluid droplets are brought into the cell using this method   _____

6. EXPLAIN WHAT WILL HAPPEN IF CELLS ARE PLACED IN SOLUTIONS WITH CONCENTRATIONS THE SAME AS OR DIFFERENT FROM THOSE OF THE CELL FLUIDS.

EXERCISE 3-7: The Effect of Osmosis on Cells (Text Fig. 3-10)

Label each of the following solutions using the term that indicates the solute concentration in the solution relative to the solute concentration in the cell.

1. _____
2. _____
3. _____

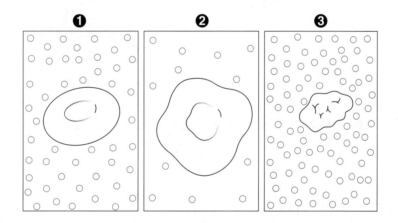

7. DESCRIBE THE COMPOSITION, LOCATION, AND FUNCTION OF THE DNA IN THE CELL.

EXERCISE 3-8: Structure of DNA
(Text Fig. 3-15)

1. Write the name of each part of the DNA molecule on the numbered lines in contrasting colors. Write the name of part 4 in the box on the diagram.
2. Color the different parts on the diagram with the corresponding color.

1. _____

2. _____

3. _____

5. _____

6. _____

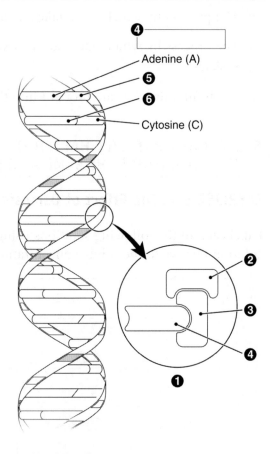

Adenine (A)

Cytosine (C)

8. COMPARE THE FUNCTION OF THREE TYPES OF RNA IN CELLS.

See Exercise 3-9.

9. EXPLAIN BRIEFLY HOW CELLS MAKE PROTEINS.

EXERCISE 3-9

Write the appropriate term in each blank from the list below.

DNA	nucleotide	transcription	ribosomal RNA (rRNA)
transfer RNA (tRNA)	messenger RNA (mRNA)	translation	

1. The process by which RNA is synthesized from the DNA _____

2. A building block of DNA and RNA _____

3. An important component of ribosomes _____

4. The structure that carries amino acids to the ribosome _____

5. The nucleic acid that carries information from the nucleus
   to the ribosomes _____

6. The process by which amino acids are assembled into a protein _____

10. NAME AND BRIEFLY DESCRIBE THE STAGES IN MITOSIS.

EXERCISE 3-10: Stages of Mitosis (Text Fig. 3-18)

Identify interphase and the indicated stages of mitosis. Find the DNA in each stage and color it.

1. _____

2. _____

3. _____

4. _____

5. _____

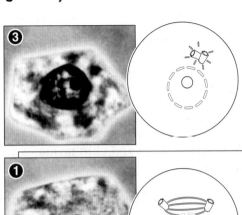
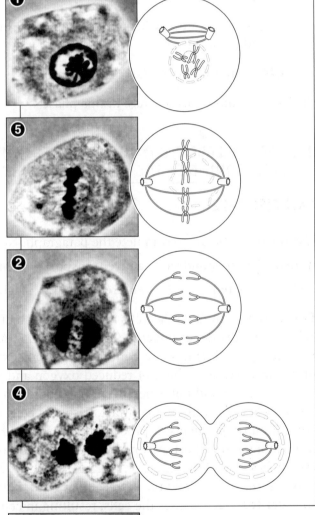
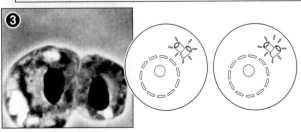

EXERCISE 3-11

Write the appropriate term in each blank from the list below.

mitosis	anaphase	telophase	meiosis
metaphase	prophase	interphase	

1. The process by which one cell divides into two identical daughter cells

   _____

2. The nuclear membrane reforms during this phase

   _____

3. A spindle begins to form and chromosomes condense during this phase

   _____

4. The phase of mitosis when chromosomes are aligned in the middle of the cell

   _____

5. DNA synthesis occurs during this phase

   _____

6. The chromosomes separate in this phase

   _____

11. USE THE CASE STUDY TO DISCUSS THE IMPORTANCE OF CELLS TO THE FUNCTIONING OF THE BODY AS A WHOLE.

EXERCISE 3-12

Use the terms below to complete the paragraph. Not all terms will be used.

mitosis	mitochondria	active transport	membrane potential
ATP	exited	entered	facilitated diffusion

Problems with Jim's cardiac cells resulted in a potentially fatal incident. First, mature cardiac muscle cells cannot divide, or undergo (1) _____. As a result, Joe's cardiac cells attempted to compensate by producing more contractile proteins within each cell. Second, Joe had a clot in one of his heart vessels. This clot reduced oxygen and glucose delivery to his cardiac cells, so the (2) _____ could not generate enough energy in the form of (3) _____. Without energy his muscle cells could not contract. Also, his cells could no longer move substances against their concentration gradients, a process described as (4) _____ _____. This disruption in membrane transport disrupted the distribution of charges across the plasma membrane, which establishes the (5) _____ _____. This disruption also altered the solute balance between the cytosol and the extracellular fluid. Solutes became more concentrated in the cytosol, so water (6) _____ the cells, resulting in cell death.

12. SHOW HOW WORD PARTS ARE USED TO BUILD WORDS RELATED TO CELLS AND THEIR FUNCTIONS.

EXERCISE 3-13

Complete the following table by writing the correct word part or meaning in the space provided. Write a word that contains each word part in the Example column.

Word Part	Meaning	Example
1. phag/o	_____	_____
2. _____	to drink	_____
3. -some	_____	_____
4. lys/o	_____	_____
5. _____	cell	_____
6. _____	above, over, excessive	_____
7. hem/o-	_____	_____
8. _____	same, equal	_____
9. hypo-	_____	_____
10. _____	in, within	_____

Making the Connections

The following concept map deals with the movement of materials through the plasma membrane. Complete the concept map by filling in the appropriate word or phrase that describes the indicated process.

1. Processes that move small quantities of material through the plasma membrane include…

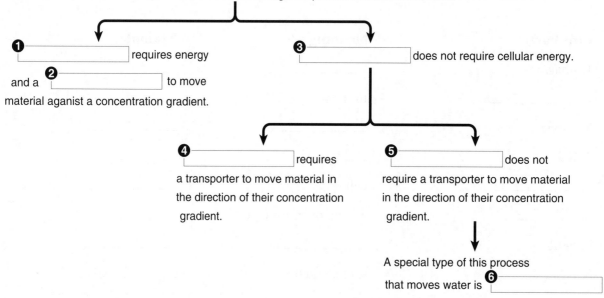

1 _____ requires energy
and a **2** _____ to move
material aganist a concentration gradient.

3 _____ does not require cellular energy.

4 _____ requires
a transporter to move material in
the direction of their concentration
gradient.

5 _____ does not
require a transporter to move material
in the direction of their concentration
gradient.

A special type of this process
that moves water is **6** _____

2. Processes that move large quantities of material through the plasma membrane include…

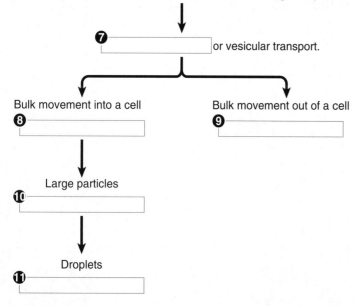

7 _____ or vesicular transport.

Bulk movement into a cell
8 _____

Bulk movement out of a cell
9 _____

Large particles
10 _____

Droplets
11 _____

Optional Exercise: Make your own concept map, based on the components of the cell. Choose your own terms to incorporate into your map, or use the following list: nucleus, mitochondria, cell membrane, protein, RNA, DNA, ATP, vesicle, ribosome, ER.

Testing Your Knowledge

BUILDING UNDERSTANDING

I. MULTIPLE CHOICE

Select the best answer and write the letter of your choice in the blank.

1. Which of the following organelles modifies proteins?
   a. mitochondrion
   b. rough endoplasmic reticulum
   c. smooth endoplasmic reticulum
   d. Golgi apparatus

1. _____

2. Which of these terms describes the process of programmed cell death?
   a. mitosis
   b. mutation
   c. apoptosis
   d. phagocytosis

2. _____

3. Which of the following are required for active transport?
   a. vesicles and cilia
   b. transporters and ATP
   c. osmotic pressure and centrioles
   d. osmosis and lysosomes

3. _____

4. During which stage of mitosis does chromatin condense into chromosomes?
   a. metaphase
   b. anaphase
   c. prophase
   d. telophase

4. _____

5. Which of these processes enables large proteins to enter the cell?
   a. active transport
   b. osmosis
   c. endocytosis
   d. exocytosis

5. _____

6. Which of these macromolecules makes up transporters, carriers, and enzymes in the plasma membrane?
   a. DNA
   b. protein
   c. carbohydrate
   d. phospholipid

6. _____

7. Which of the following tools has the greatest magnification?
   a. scanning electron microscope
   b. transmission electron microscope
   c. light microscope
   d. magnifying glass

7. _____

8. Which of these terms describes a solution that causes cells to
   shrink when they are placed in it?   8. _____
      a. isotonic
      b. hypotonic
      c. hypertonic
      d. osmotic

II. COMPLETION EXERCISE

Write the word or phrase that correctly completes each sentence.

1. The most abundant cation (positively charged ion) in the extracellular fluid is

   _____.

2. The plasma membrane contains two kinds of lipids: cholesterol and

   _____.

3. The single small dark body within the nucleus is called the _____.

4. The four nitrogen bases found in DNA are A, T, G, and _____.

5. The four nitrogen bases found in RNA are A, C, G, and _____.

6. The assembly of an RNA strand is called _____.

7. The type of RNA that carries individual amino acids is called _____.

8. The chromosomes duplicate during the period between mitoses, which is called

   _____.

9. A cell has four chromosomes before entering the process of mitosis. After mitosis, the number of chromosomes in each daughter cell will be _____.

10. Transporters are used for the processes of active transport and _____.

11. Droplets of water and dissolved substances are brought into the cell by the process of

    _____.

12. Water crosses plasma membranes through specialized channels called

    _____.

13. Bacteria are brought into the cell by the process of _____.

UNDERSTANDING CONCEPTS

I. TRUE/FALSE

For each question, write T for true or F for false in the blank to the left of each number. If a statement is false, correct it by replacing the underlined term and write the correct statement in the blanks below the question.

_____ 1. The nucleotide sequence "ACCTG" would be found in <u>DNA</u>.

_____

_____ 2. A living cell (with a tonicity equivalent to 0.9% NaCl) is placed in a solution containing 0.2% NaCl. This solution is <u>hypertonic</u>.

_____

_____ 3. Glucose is moving into a cell, down its concentration gradient, using a carrier protein. Glucose is traveling by <u>active transport</u>.

_____

_____ 4. A toxin has entered a cell. The cell is no longer capable of generating ATP. The most likely explanation for this effect is that the toxin has destroyed the <u>mitochondria</u>.

_____

_____ 5. The passage of water and dissolved materials through a membrane under pressure is called <u>osmosis</u>.

_____

_____ 6. It is impossible to count individual chromosomes during <u>interphase</u>.

_____

II. PRACTICAL APPLICATIONS

Study each discussion. Then write the appropriate word or phrase in the space provided. The following are observations you might make while working for the summer in a hospital laboratory.

1. A sample of breast tissue that was thought to be cancerous arrived at the hospital laboratory. The milk-producing cells of the breast produce large amounts of protein. The small RNA-containing bodies that synthesize proteins are called _____.

2. The tissue was in a liquid called normal saline so that the cells would neither shrink nor swell. Normal saline contains 0.9% salt, and is thus considered to be

   _____.

3. The pathologist (Dr. C) sliced the tissue very thinly and placed it on a microscope slide, but he was unable to see anything. Unfortunately, he had forgotten to add a dye to the tissue. These special dyes are called _____.

4. Dr. C went back to his bench in order to get the necessary dye. He noticed that there were many impurities floating in the dye, and he decided to screen them out. He separated the solid particles from the liquid by forcing the liquid through a membrane, a process called

   _____.

5. Dr. C was clumsy and accidentally spilled the dye into a sink full of dishes. The water in the sink rapidly turned pink. The dye molecules had moved through the water by the process of _____.

6. Dr. C made up some new dye and treated the tissue. Finally, the tissue was ready for examination. Which type of microscope uses light to view stained tissues? _____.

7. The pathologist looked at the tissue and noticed that the nuclei of many cells were in the process of dividing. This division process is called _____.

8. Some cells were in the stage of cell division called prophase. The DNA was condensed into structures called _____.

9. Dr. C sent a sample to a laboratory that specialized in identifying alterations in gene structure. The technicians in this laboratory identified a change in the sequence of a specific gene called the BRCA-1 gene. In place of an A nucleotide, there was the nucleotide than normally pairs with cytosine (C). This nucleotide is abbreviated as _____.

III. SHORT ESSAYS

1. Compare and contrast active transport and facilitated diffusion. List at least 1 similarity and at least 1 difference.

   _____

   _____

   _____

   _____

   _____

2. You are in the hospital for a minor operation, and the technician is hooking you up to an IV. He knows you are a biology student and jokingly asks if you would like a hypertonic, hypotonic, or isotonic solution to be placed in your IV. Which solution would you pick? Explain your answer.

   _____

   _____

   _____

   _____

   _____

3. List the four stages of mitosis and briefly describe each.

_____

_____

_____

_____

_____

CONCEPTUAL THINKING

1. Compare the structure of a cell to a factory or a city. Try to find cell structures that accomplish all of the different functions of the city or a factory.

_____

_____

_____

_____

_____

2. Your great-aunt M is 96 years old and loves to hear about what you are learning in class. She recently attended an Elderhostel camp, where people were talking about this new-fangled notion called DNA.
   a. She asks you to explain why DNA is so important. Explain the role of DNA in protein synthesis, using clear, uncomplicated language. You must define any term that your Great-aunt might not know. You can use an analogy if you like.

_____

_____

_____

_____

   b. Next, your great-aunt wonders how the proteins get out of the cell. Explain the pathway a protein takes from the ribosome to the blood. You can use an illustration if you like.

_____

_____

_____

_____

3. You are a xenobiologist studying an alien cell isolated on Mars. Surprisingly, you notice that the cell contains some of the same substances as our cells. You quantify the concentration of these substances and determine that the cell contains 10% glucose and 0.3% calcium. The cell is placed in a solution containing 20% glucose and 0.1% calcium. The plasma membrane of this cell is very different to ours. It is permeable to glucose but not to calcium. That is, only glucose can cross the plasma membrane without using transporters. Use this information to answer the following questions:

a. Will glucose move into the cell or out of the cell? Which transport mechanism will be involved?

_____

_____

b. Carrier proteins are present in the membrane that can transport calcium. If calcium moves down its concentration gradient, will calcium move into the cell or out of the cell? Which transport mechanism will be involved?

_____

_____

c. You place the cell in a new solution to study the process of osmosis. You know that sodium does not move across the alien cell membrane. You also know that the concentration of the intracellular fluid is equivalent to 1% sodium. The new solution contains 2% sodium.

(i) Is the 2% sodium solution hypertonic, isotonic, or hypotonic?

_____

(ii) Will water flow into the cell or out of the cell? _____

(iii) What will be the effect of the water movement on cell volume?

_____

Expanding Your Horizons

Thanks to the Human Genome Project, we now know the DNA sequence of every human gene. Imagine some of the possibilities this information presents—we can screen for susceptibility to cancer and diabetes, and maybe, just maybe, find out about the potential intelligence, height, and sports abilities of our babies before they are even born. These possibilities raise all kinds of ethical dilemmas. Will genetic screening soon be required to obtain health insurance? Will some parents use prenatal screening to select for a superbaby? How can we keep genetic information secure from computer hackers? The articles listed below provide more information.

- Aldhous P, Reilly M. How my Genome was hacked. New Sci 2009;201:6–9.
- Hall SS. Revolution postponed. Sci Am 2010;303:60–67.

CHAPTER

4

Tissues, Glands, and Membranes

Overview

The cell is the basic unit of life. Individual cells are grouped according to function into **tissues**. The four main groups of tissues include **epithelial tissue**, which forms glands, covers surfaces, and lines cavities; **connective tissue**, which gives support and form to the body; **muscle tissue**, which produces movement; and **nervous tissue**, which conducts electrical impulses.

All tissues derive from **stem cells**, actively dividing cells whose offspring can remain as stem cells or differentiate into specialized tissue cells. Small stem cell populations persist into adulthood so that tissues can renew and repair themselves. Glands produce substances used by other cells and tissues. **Exocrine glands** produce secretions that are released through ducts to nearby parts of the body. **Endocrine glands** produce hormones that are carried by the blood to all parts of the body.

The simplest combination of tissues is a **membrane**. Membranes serve several purposes, a few of which are mentioned here: they may serve as dividing partitions, may line hollow organs and cavities, and may anchor various organs. Membranes that have epithelial cells on the surface are referred to as **epithelial membranes**. Two types of epithelial membranes are **serous membranes**, which line body cavities and cover the internal organs, and **mucous membranes**, which line passageways leading to the outside.

The study of tissues, known as **histology**, requires much memorization. In particular, you may be challenged to learn the different types of epithelial and connective tissue as well as the classification scheme of epithelial and connective membranes. Learning the structure of these different tissues and membranes will help you understand the amazing properties of the body, such as how we can jump from great heights, swim without becoming waterlogged, and fold our ears over without breaking them.

Addressing the Learning Outcomes

1. NAME THE FOUR MAIN GROUPS OF TISSUES AND GIVE THE LOCATION AND GENERAL CHARACTERISTICS OF EACH.

EXERCISE 4-1: Four Types of Epithelium (Text Fig. 4-1)

Label each of the following types of epithelium.

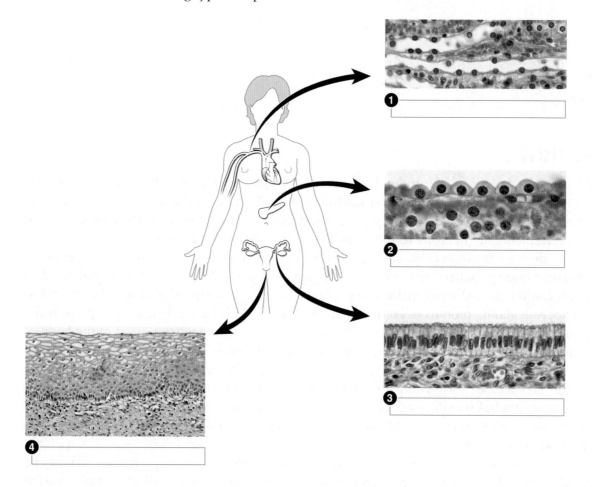

EXERCISE 4-2: Muscle Tissue (Text Fig. 4-6)

Write the names of the three types of muscle tissue in the appropriate blanks in different colors. Color some of the muscle cells the appropriate color. Look for the nuclei, and color them a different color.

1. _____

2. _____

3. _____

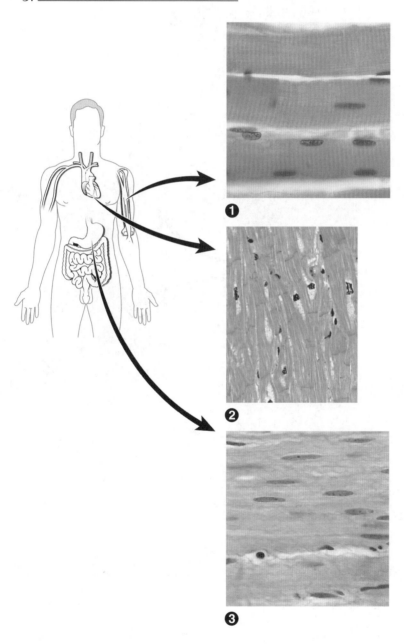

EXERCISE 4-3: Nervous Tissue (Text Fig. 4-7)

1. Write the names of each tissue (indicating the plane of the section where appropriate) in boxes 7 to 9.
2. Label each of the following neural structures and tissues using different colors. Where possible, color each structure or tissue with the appropriate color.

1. _____

2. _____

3. _____

4. _____

5. _____

6. _____

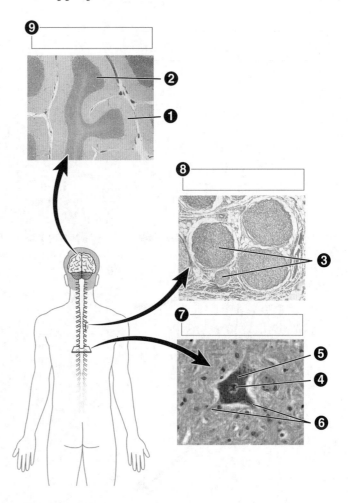

EXERCISE 4-4

Write the appropriate term in each blank from the list below.

tissue   squamous   stratified   transitional
cuboidal   columnar   simple

1. A group of cells similar in structure and function   _____

2. Term that describes flat, irregular epithelial cells   _____

3. A term that means *in layers*   _____

4. Term that describes long and narrow epithelial cells   _____

5. Term that describes square epithelial cells   _____

6. Cells arranged in a single layer   _____

EXERCISE 4-5

Write the appropriate term in each blank from the list below.

bone   myocardium   voluntary muscle   epithelial tissue

neuron   smooth muscle   neuroglia   connective tissue

1. The thigh muscle is an example of   _____

2. Tissue that forms when cartilage gradually becomes
   impregnated with calcium salts   _____

3. The thick, muscular layer of the heart wall   _____

4. A type of tissue found in membrane and glands   _____

5. Visceral muscle is also known as   _____

6. A cell that carries nerve impulses is called a(n)   _____

7. A tissue in which cells are separated by large amounts of
   acellular material called matrix   _____

2. DESCRIBE THE DIFFERENCE BETWEEN EXOCRINE AND ENDOCRINE GLANDS AND GIVE EXAMPLES OF EACH.

EXERCISE 4-6

Fill in the blank after each statement—does it apply to exocrine glands (EX), endocrine glands (EN), or both (B)?

1. A gland that secretes into the blood _____

2. A gland that secretes through ducts _____

3. A gland that secretes onto the body surface _____

4. The pituitary gland, for example _____

5. A group of cells that produces substances for use by other parts of the body _____

6. Salivary glands, for example _____

3. GIVE EXAMPLES OF CIRCULATING, GENERALIZED, AND STRUCTURAL CONNECTIVE TISSUES.

EXERCISE 4-7: Connective Tissue (Text Figs. 4-4 and 4-5)

Write the names of the six examples of connective tissue in the appropriate boxes. Use red for the circulating connective tissue (1), three different shades of green for the generalized tissues (2–4), and two shades of blue for the structural tissues (5–6). Color some of the **cells** of each tissue type with the corresponding color.

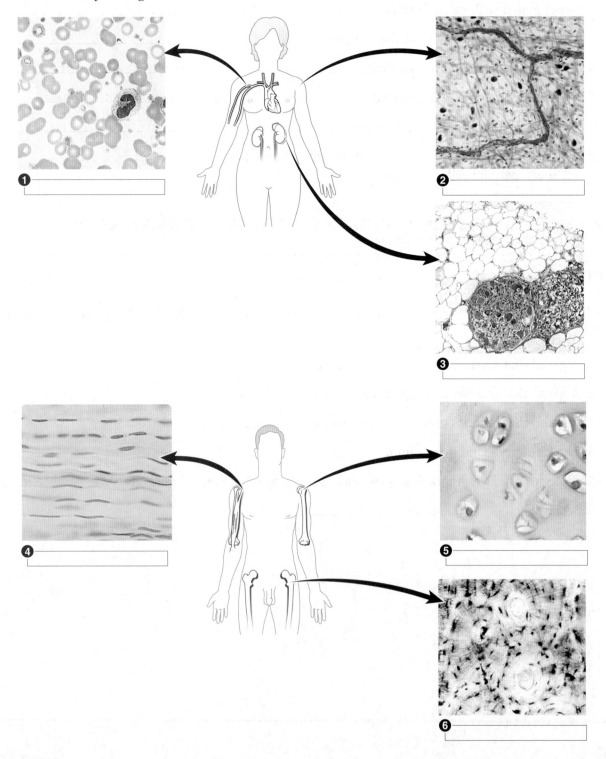

EXERCISE 4-8

Write the appropriate term in each blank from the list below.

ligament   tendon   collagen   chondrocyte

capsule   hyaline cartilage   elastic cartilage   fibrocartilage

1. A cord of connective tissue that connects a muscle to a bone   _____

2. A tough membranous connective tissue that encloses an organ   _____

3. The cartilage found between the bones of the spine   _____

4. A fiber found in most connective tissues   _____

5. A cell that synthesizes cartilage   _____

6. A strong, gristly cartilage that reinforces the trachea   _____

4. DESCRIBE THREE TYPES OF EPITHELIAL MEMBRANES.

EXERCISE 4-9

Write the appropriate term in each blank from the list below.

mesothelium   serous membrane   cutaneous membrane   parietal layer

visceral layer   mucous membrane   peritoneum   serous pericardium

1. An epithelial membrane that lines a body cavity or covers an internal organ   _____

2. The epithelial membrane also known as the skin   _____

3. A membrane that lines a space open to the outside of the body   _____

4. The portion of a serous membrane attached to an organ   _____

5. The portion of a serous membrane attached to the body wall   _____

6. The epithelial portion of serous membranes   _____

7. The serous membrane covering the heart   _____

5. LIST SEVERAL TYPES OF CONNECTIVE TISSUE MEMBRANES.

EXERCISE 4-10

Write the appropriate term in each blank from the list below.

periosteum	fibrous pericardium	perichondrium	epithelial membrane
synovial membrane	superficial fascia	deep fascia	connective tissue membrane

1. The sheet of tissue that underlies the skin _____

2. The connective tissue membrane that lines joint cavities _____

3. A tough membrane composed entirely of connective tissue that serves to anchor and support an organ or to cover a muscle _____

4. A layer of fibrous connective tissue around a bone _____

5. The membrane that covers cartilage _____

6. A general term describing a membrane composed of epithelial and connective tissue _____

7. A general term describing a membrane composed exclusively of connective tissue _____

6. USING THE CASE STUDY, DESCRIBE THE CONSEQUENCE OF TISSUE CHANGES ON ORGANS AND SYSTEMS.

EXERCISE 4-11

Fill in the blanks in the paragraph using the terms in the list. You will not use all of the terms. Some answers require two terms (such as "simple" and "cuboidal").

cystic fibrosis	simple	pseudostratified	stratified
columnar	cuboidal	squamous	epidermis

Ben, the subject of the case study, suffered from a genetic disease called (1) _____ _____. In this disease, a faulty chloride channel impacts the functioning of many epithelial membranes. For instance, the ducts lining his pancreas were blocked. These ducts are lined with a single layer of square cells, known as (2) _____ _____ epithelium. His respiratory passages were similarly blocked. The largest of these tubes are lined with a single layer of tall, thin cells that appears to consist of multiple layers. This type of epithelial membrane contains (3) _____ _____ epithelium. Ben's diagnosis was aided by secretions from the epithelial membrane of his skin, known as the (4) _____. This membrane consists of (5) _____ _____ epithelium since it contains many layers of flattened cells.

Testing Your Knowledge

BUILDING UNDERSTANDING

I. MULTIPLE CHOICE

Select the best answer and write the letter of your choice in the blank.

1. Which of the following is a type of connective tissue?
   a. transitional
   b. squamous
   c. cuboidal
   d. areolar

1. _____

2. Which of these phrases describes simple cuboidal epithelium?
   a. flat, irregular, epithelial cells in a single layer
   b. square epithelial cells in a single layer
   c. long, narrow, epithelial cells in a single layer
   d. square epithelial cells in many layers

2. _____

3. Which muscle type is under voluntary control?
   a. smooth muscle
   b. skeletal muscle
   c. cardiac muscle
   d. visceral muscle

3. _____

4. What is the proper scientific name for a nerve cell?
   a. neuroglia
   b. nevus
   c. neuron
   d. axon

4. _____

5. Which cell type secretes mucus?
   a. endocrine
   b. goblet
   c. areolar
   d. fibroblast

5. _____

6. Which cell type produces cartilage?
   a. chondrocytes
   b. fibroblasts
   c. osteoblasts
   d. osteocytes

6. _____

7. Which of these tissues is an example of loose connective tissue?
   a. ligament
   b. adipose
   c. tendon
   d. bone

7. _____

8. What is the tough connective tissue membrane that covers most parts of all bones?
   a. perichondrium
   b. periosteum
   c. fascia
   d. ligament

8. _____

9. Which of these phrases describes the membrane surrounding skeletal muscles ?

    9. _____

    a. deep fascia
    b. fibrous pericardium
    c. superficial fascia
    d. perichondrium

II. COMPLETION EXERCISE

Write the word or phrase that correctly completes each sentence.

1. The secretion that traps dust and other inhaled particles is called _____.

2. Cells that form bone are called _____.

3. The cartilage found at the end of long bones is called _____.

4. The connective tissue membrane lining joint cavities is called the _____.

5. The study of tissues is called _____.

6. The epithelial membrane that lines the walls of the abdominal cavity is called the _____.

7. A mucous membrane can also be called the _____.

8. A single layer of flat, irregular epithelial cells is called _____.

9. The microscopic, hairlike projections found in the cells lining most of the respiratory tract are called _____.

UNDERSTANDING CONCEPTS

I. TRUE/FALSE

For each question, write T for true or F for false in the blank to the left of each number. If a statement is false, correct it by replacing the underlined term and write the correct statement in the blanks below the question.

_____ 1. The peritoneum is an example of a mucous membrane.

_____

_____ 2. The strip of tissue connecting the kneecap to the thigh muscle is an example of a tendon.

_____

_____ 3. The periosteum is a connective tissue membrane surrounding bone.

_____

_____ 4. The pituitary gland releases prolactin into the bloodstream. The pituitary gland is thus an <u>exocrine</u> gland.

_____

_____ 5. The <u>parietal</u> layer of the peritoneum is in contact with the stomach.

_____

_____ 6. Ligaments are classified as <u>irregular loose connective tissue</u>.

_____

II. PRACTICAL APPLICATIONS

Study each discussion. Then write the appropriate word or phrase in the space provided.

You are working as a sports therapist for a wrestling team. At a particularly brutal competition, you are asked to evaluate a number of injuries.

1. Mr. K suffered a crushing injury to the lower leg yesterday in a sumo wrestling match when his opponent fell on him. Initially, he had little pain. Now, he complains of numbness and pain in the foot and leg. This type of injury is made worse by the tight, fibrous covering of the muscles, known as the _____.

2. Mr. K is also complaining of pain in the knee. You suspect an injury to the membrane that lines the joint cavity, a membrane called the _____.

3. You note that Mr. K has a significant amount of fat. Fat is contained in a type of connective tissue called _____.

4. Based on its consistency, this tissue is classified as _____.

5. Ms. J suffered a painful bump on her ankle. The swelling involved the superficial tissues and the fibrous covering of the bone, or the _____.

6. Mr. S was involved in a closely fought match when his opponent bent his ear back. Thankfully, the cartilage in his ear was able to spring back into shape. This kind of cartilage is called _____.

7. Later, Mr. S suffered a penetrating wound to his abdomen when his opponent accidentally threw him into the seating area. You fear that the wound may have penetrated the membrane that lines his abdomen, called the _____.

8. The wrestling coach comes over to talk to you during a break in the match. He has a question about his favorite shampoo. The advertisement stated that it contained collagen. He asks you which cells in the body synthesize collagen. These cells are called _____.

III. SHORT ESSAYS

1. Compare and contrast epithelial tissue membranes and give an example of each. List at least one similarity and one difference in your answer.

   _____

   _____

   _____

   _____

   _____

2. Differentiate between epithelial tissue, connective tissue, and muscle in terms of the amount and composition of the extracellular matrix.

   _____

   _____

   _____

   _____

   _____

CONCEPTUAL THINKING

1. Why are bone and blood both considered to be connective tissue? Define connective tissue in your answer.

   _____

   _____

   _____

   _____

   _____

2. Which tissue, epithelial or connective, would be best suited to the following functions?
   a. cushioning the kidneys against a blow.

   _____

   b. creating a virtually waterproof barrier between the body and the environment

   _____

   c. preventing toxins from entering the blood from the gastrointestinal tract

   _____

3. A number of the components of a joint are listed below. Name the tissue type and/or membrane for each. Provide as many descriptive terms as you can. For instance, the tissue in the vocal cords can be classified as elastic connective tissue and generalized connective tissue.
    a. the ends of the bones are covered with tough, translucent cartilage

    _____

    b. a fluid-secreting membrane secretes synovial fluid

    _____

    c. small fat pads cushion the joint

    _____

    d. tendons pass over the joint and contribute to the strength of the joint

    _____

    e. ligaments bind the bones together

    _____

Expanding Your Horizons

Text Box 4-1 talks about some of the possibilities and ethical dilemmas surrounding stem cell use. Although stem cells have enormous potential, the technical and political difficulties involved sometimes seem insumountable. Indeed, it has proved difficult to find true stem cells that can differentiate into any cell type. Many alleged stem cell lines can only produce certain types of cells. Much research remains to be done regarding techniques to identify stem cells and the factors that cause differentiation into different cell types. You can learn more about the politics, difficulties, and potential of stem cell research in the following article.

- Lanza R, Rosenthal N. The stem cell challenge. Sci Am 2004;290:92–100.

CHAPTER 5

The Integumentary System

Overview

Because of its various properties, the skin can be classified as a membrane, an organ, or a system. The outermost layer of the skin is the **epidermis**. Beneath the epidermis is the **dermis** (the true skin) where glands and other accessory structures are mainly located. The **subcutaneous tissue** underlies the skin. It contains fat that serves as insulation. The accessory structures of the skin are the **sudoriferous** (sweat) **glands**, the oil-secreting **sebaceous glands**, **hair**, and **nails**.

The skin protects deeper tissues against drying and against invasion by harmful organisms. It regulates body temperature through evaporation of sweat and loss of heat at the surface. It collects information from the environment by means of sensory receptors.

The protein **keratin** in the epidermis thickens and protects the skin and makes up hair and nails. **Melanin** is the main pigment that gives the skin its color. It functions to filter out harmful ultraviolet radiation from the sun. Skin color is also influenced by the quantity and oxygen content of blood circulating in the surface blood vessels.

This chapter does not contain any particularly difficult material. However, you must be familiar with the different tissue types discussed in Chapter 4 in order to understand the structure and function of the skin and associated glands.

Addressing the Learning Outcomes

1. NAME AND DESCRIBE THE LAYERS OF THE SKIN.

EXERCISE 5-1

Write the appropriate term in each blank from the list below.

melanocyte	integument	keratin	dermis	epidermis
stratum corneum	dermal papillae	stratum basale	subcutaneous layer	

1. A pigment-producing cell that becomes more active in the presence of ultraviolet light   _____

2. The protein in the epidermis that thickens and protects the skin   _____

3. The deeper of the two major layers of skin   _____

4. The uppermost epidermal layer, consisting of flat, keratin-filled cells   _____

5. Another name for the skin as a whole   _____

6. Projections of the dermis responsible for fingerprints   _____

7. The deepest layer of the epidermis, which contains living, dividing cells   _____

8. Another name for the superficial fascia   _____

2. DESCRIBE THE SUBCUTANEOUS TISSUE.

EXERCISE 5-2

Match the structures in the list below with their functions by writing the appropriate term in each blank.

adipose tissue   elastic fibers   blood vessels   nerves

1. Connect the subcutaneous tissue with the dermis   _____

2. Insulates the body and acts as an energy reserve   _____

3. Carry sensory information from the skin to the brain   _____

4. Supply skin with nutrients and oxygen   _____

3. GIVE THE LOCATION AND THE FUNCTION OF THE ACCESSORY STRUCTURES OF THE INTEGUMENTARY SYSTEM.

EXERCISE 5-3

Write the appropriate term in each blank from the list below.

apocrine   eccrine   ceruminous   sudoriferous   wax

vernix caseosa   sebaceous   sebum   meibomian

1. A general term for any gland that produces sweat   _____

2. Sweat glands found throughout the skin that help cool the body   _____

3. Glands that are found only in the ear canal   _____

4. Excess activity of these glands contributes to acne vulgaris   _____

5. The product of ceruminous glands   _____

6. Sweat glands in the armpits and groin that become active at puberty   _____

7. Glands that lubricate the eye   _____

8. A secretion of sebaceous glands that covers newborn babies   _____

EXERCISE 5-4: The Skin (Text Fig. 5-1)

1. Write the names of the three skin layers in the numbered boxes 1 to 3.
2. On the next page, write the name of each labeled part on the numbered lines in different colors. Use a light color for structures 4 and 12. Use the same color for structures 15 and 16, for structures 13 and 14, and for structures 8 and 9.
3. Color the different structures on the diagram with the corresponding color. Try to color every structure in the figure with the appropriate color. For instance, structure number 8 is found in three locations.

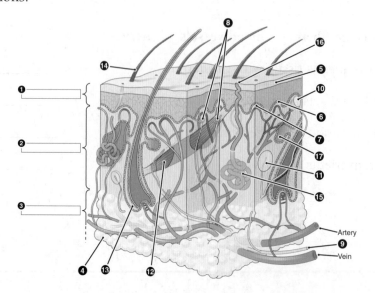

4. _____	11. _____
5. _____	12. _____
6. _____	13. _____
7. _____	14. _____
8. _____	15. _____
9. _____	16. _____
10. _____	17. _____

EXERCISE 5-5: The Nail (Text Fig. 5-5)

1. In the middle column of the table, write the name of the labeled structure.
2. In the right-hand column of the table, write a brief description of the structure.

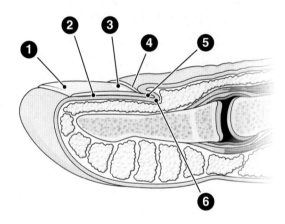

Number	Structure	Description
1.		
2.		
3.		
4.		
5.		
6.		

4. LIST THE MAIN FUNCTIONS OF THE INTEGUMENTARY SYSTEM.

EXERCISE 5-6

Fill in the numbered blanks of the table below.

Function	Structures Involved
(1)	Stratum corneum, shedding skin cells
Protection against dehydration	(2)
Regulation of body temperature	(3)
(4)	Nerve endings, specialized receptors

5. DISCUSS THE FACTORS THAT CONTRIBUTE TO SKIN COLOR.

EXERCISE 5-7

Write the appropriate term in each blank from the list below.

carotene   hemoglobin   melanin

1. The pigment that gives blood its color   _____

2. A pigment found in some vegetables that is stored in adipose tissue   _____

3. The pigment that helps protect against UV radiation   _____

6. USING INFORMATION IN THE CASE STUDY AND TEXT, DESCRIBE THE SPECIFIC LAYER OF THE INTEGUMENTARY SYSTEM THAT WAS SUN-DAMAGED.

EXERCISE 5-8

Fill in the blanks in the following description of Paul's tumor, surgery, and healing, using these terms: cicatrix, blood clot, fibroblasts, epidermis, capillaries, inflammatory response, collagen.

In Paul's case, repeated exposure to ultraviolet rays in sunlight damaged the outermost of two main skin layers, the (1) _____. Surgery removed the tumor, creating a wound. After a skin wound, the first responses are the formation of a (2) _____ _____ to stanch the bleeding and the development of an (3) _____ _____ that makes the tissue swollen and red. Tissue repair involves the formation of new (4) _____ to bring blood to the new tissue and the production of a protein called (5) _____ by connective tissue cells called (6) _____. Sometimes, the damage is too extensive for complete repair, so the tissue is replaced by connective tissue that forms a scar, or (7) _____.

7. SHOW HOW WORD PARTS ARE USED TO BUILD WORDS RELATED TO THE INTEGUMENTARY SYSTEM.

EXERCISE 5-9

Complete the following table by writing the correct word part or meaning in the space provided. Write a word that contains each word part in the Example column.

Word Part	Meaning	Example
1. sub-	_____	_____
2. _____	dark, black	_____
3. hair	_____	_____
4. dermat/o	_____	_____
5. _____	cornified, keratinized	_____
6. ap/o-	_____	_____

Making the Connections

The following concept map deals with the structural features of the skin. Complete the concept map by filling in the appropriate word or phrase in each box.

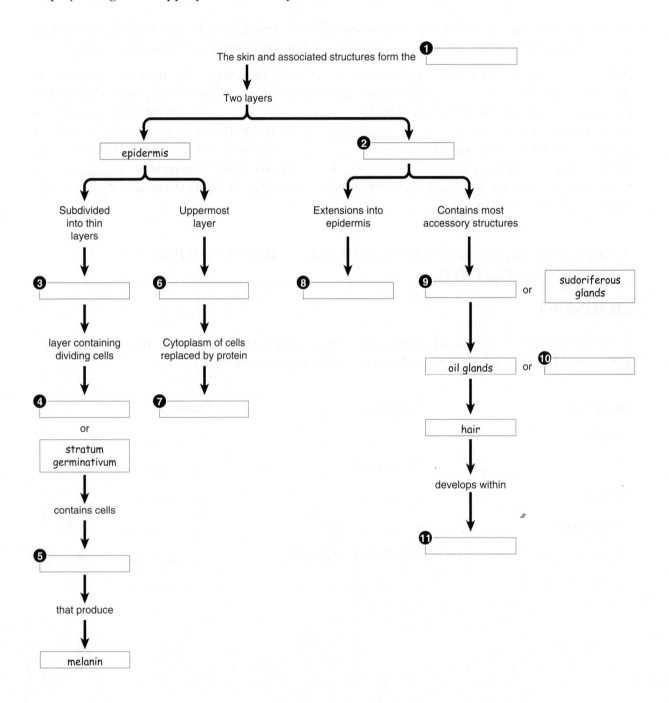

Testing Your Knowledge

BUILDING UNDERSTANDING

I. MULTIPLE CHOICE

Select the best answer and write the letter of your choice in the blank.

1. Where are new epidermal cells produced?
   a. dermis
   b. stratum corneum
   c. stratum basale
   d. subcutaneous layer

   1. _____

2. Which of the following glands is NOT a modified sweat gland?
   a. mammary gland
   b. sebaceous gland
   c. ceruminous gland
   d. ciliary gland

   2. _____

3. Which term describes a narrowing of a blood vessel?
   a. dilation
   b. constriction
   c. closure
   d. merger

   3. _____

4. What is the white half-moon at the base of the nail called?
   a. root
   b. matrix
   c. lunula
   d. cuticle

   4. _____

5. Which of these glands produces ear wax?
   a. ciliary gland
   b. ceruminous gland
   c. sudoriferous gland
   d. eccrine gland

   5. _____

6. What is the name of the muscle connected to hair follicles?
   a. ciliary muscle
   b. arrector pili
   c. sebaceous muscle
   d. vernix

   6. _____

II. COMPLETION EXERCISE

Write the word or phrase that correctly completes each sentence.

1. The outer layer of the epidermis, which contains flat, keratin-filled cells, is called the

   _____.

2. Fingerprints are created by extensions of the dermis into the epidermis. These extensions are called _____.

3. The main pigment of the skin is _____.

4. The cells that secrete collagen to help close a wound are called _____.

5. The subcutaneous layer is also called the hypodermis or the _____.

6. The ceruminous glands and the ciliary glands are modified forms of _____.

7. Hair and nails are composed mainly of a protein named _____.

UNDERSTANDING CONCEPTS

I. TRUE/FALSE

For each question, write T for true or F for false in the blank to the left of each number. If a statement is false, correct it by replacing the underlined term and write the correct statement in the blanks below the question.

_____ 1. The nail cuticle, which seals the space between the nail plate and the skin above the nail root, is an extension of the stratum basale.

_____

_____ 2. In cold weather, the blood vessels in the skin constrict in order to conserve heat.

_____

_____ 3. The skin produces vitamin A under the influence of ultraviolet light.

_____

_____ 4. Sebum is produced by sudoriferous glands.

_____

_____ 5. The part of the hair below the skin surface is the follicle.

_____

_____ 6. The stratum corneum is the deepest layer of the epidermis.

_____

II. PRACTICAL APPLICATIONS

Study each discussion. Then write the appropriate word or phrase in the space provided.

Mr B has suffered a fall in a downhill mountain biking competition. Working as a first-aid volunteer, you are the first person arriving at the scene of the accident.

1. Mr B has light scratches on his left cheek. The scratches are not bleeding, indicating that they have only penetrated the uppermost layer of the epidermis, known as the _____.

2. A branch tore a long jagged wound in his right arm. This wound has penetrated into the tissue underneath the dermis, known as the superficial fascia or _____.

3. The skin of Mr B's nose is very brown. The brown color reflects the presence of a pigment called _____.

4. Mr B has difficulties hearing your questions. You examine his ears and discover that they are full of ear wax. Ear wax is synthesized by modified sweat glands called

   _____.

5. You note that Mr B has a rather strong body odor. Body odor reflects the secretions of glands called _____.

6. When you examine Mr B, you see numerous healed wounds. These wounds were healed through the actions of cells called _____.

7. The new tissue that healed the wound is called a scar, or a _____.

8. Mr B, like many young men, suffers from acne vulgaris. This skin disease, which is characterized by pimples and blackheads, involves infection of the oil-producing glands of the skin called the _____.

III. SHORT ESSAYS

1. Compare and contrast eccrine and apocrine sweat (sudoriferous) glands.

   _____

   _____

   _____

2. Describe the role that the skin plays in the regulation of body temperature.

   _____

   _____

   _____

CONCEPTUAL THINKING

1. Describe the location and structure of the different tissue types (epithelial, muscle, nervous, connective) present in the integumentary system.

   _____

   _____

   _____

   _____

2. Discuss the functional implications of the following structural changes in skin associated with aging.

a. less subcutaneous fat and decreased circulation in the dermis

_____

_____

b. decreased melanin production in hair and skin

_____

_____

c. decreased cell proliferation in the hair follicle

_____

_____

d. reduced collagen and elastic production in the dermis

_____

_____

e. decreased activity of the eccrine sudoriferous glands

_____

_____

Expanding Your Horizons

Why did different skin tones evolve? It is often thought that darker pigmentation (more melanin) has evolved to protect humans from skin cancer. However, since skin cancer occurs later in life (usually postreproductive age), it cannot exert much evolutionary pressure. The advantages and disadvantages of darker skin tone are discussed in these *Scientific American* articles:

- Jablonski NG, Chaplin G. Skin deep. Sci Am 2002;287:74–81.
- Tavera-Mendoza LE, White JH. Cell defenses and the sunshine vitamin. Sci Am 2007;(November):62–72.

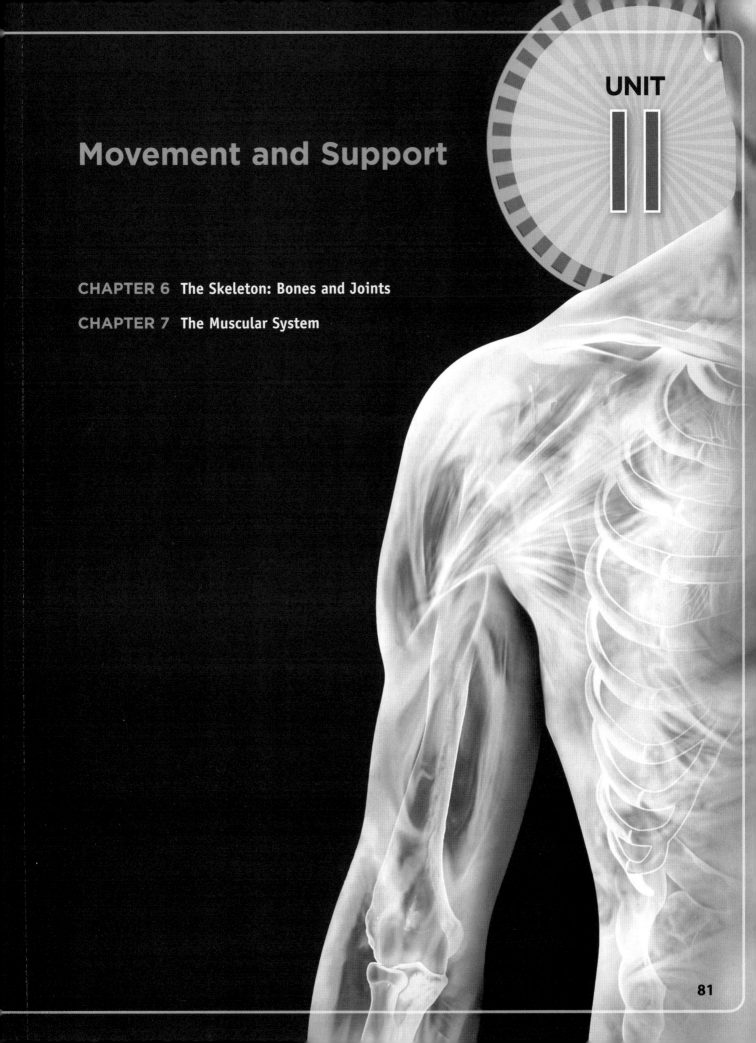

Movement and Support

UNIT

II

CHAPTER
6

The Skeleton: Bones and Joints

Overview

The skeletal system protects and supports the body parts and serves as attachment points for the muscles, which furnish the power for movement. The bones also store calcium salts and are the site of blood cell production. The skeletal system includes some 206 bones; the number varies slightly according to age and the individual.

Although bone tissue contains a matrix of nonliving material, bones also contain living cells and have their own systems of blood vessels and nerves. Bone tissue may be either **spongy** or **compact**. Compact bone is found in the **diaphysis** (shaft) of long bones and in the outer layer of other bones. Spongy bone makes up the **epiphyses** (ends) of long bones and the center of other bones. **Red marrow**, present at the ends of long bones and the center of other bones, manufactures blood cells; **yellow marrow**, which is largely fat, is found in the central (medullary) cavities of the long bones.

Bone tissue is produced by cells called **osteoblasts**, which gradually convert cartilage to bone during development and add bone tissue for remodeling and repair throughout life. The mature cells that maintain bone are called **osteocytes**, and the cells that break down (resorb) bone for remodeling and repair are the **osteoclasts**.

The skeleton is divided into two main groups of bones, the **axial skeleton** and the **appendicular skeleton**. The axial skeleton includes the skull, spinal column, ribs, and sternum. The appendicular skeleton consists of the bones of the upper and lower extremities, the shoulder girdle, and the pelvic girdle.

A **joint** is the region of union of two or more bones. Joints are classified into three main types on the basis of the material between the connecting bones. In **fibrous joints**, the bones are held together by fibrous connective tissue, and in **cartilaginous joints**, the bones are joined by cartilage. In **synovial joints**, the material between the bones is synovial fluid, which is secreted by the synovial membrane lining the joint cavity. The bones in synovial joints are connected by ligaments. Synovial joints show the greatest degree of movement, and the six types of synovial joints allow for a variety of movements in different directions.

Addressing the Learning Outcomes

1. LIST THE FUNCTIONS OF BONES.

EXERCISE 6-1

List five functions of bones in the spaces provided.

1. _____

2. _____

3. _____

4. _____

5. _____

2. DESCRIBE THE STRUCTURE OF A LONG BONE.

EXERCISE 6-2: Structure of a Long Bone (Text Fig. 6-2)

1. Write the names of the three parts of a long bone in the numbered boxes 1–3.
2. Write the name of each labeled part on the numbered lines in different colors. Use a dark color for structure 5.
3. Color the different structures on the diagram with the corresponding color.

4. _____

5. _____

6. _____

7. _____

8. _____

9. _____

10. _____

11. _____

12. _____

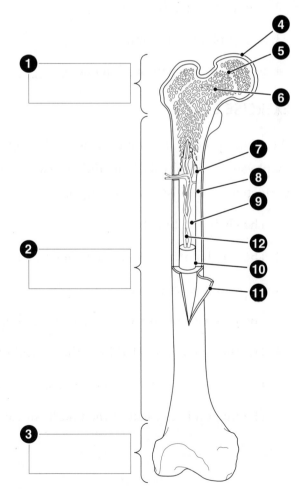

3. DIFFERENTIATE BETWEEN COMPACT BONE AND SPONGY BONE WITH RESPECT TO STRUCTURE AND LOCATION.

EXERCISE 6-3

Fill in the blank after each statement—does it apply to compact bone (C) or spongy bone (S)?

1. Makes up the interior of the epiphyses of long bones _____

2. Makes up the center of short bones_____

3. Makes up the shaft of a long bone _____

4. A meshwork of small, bony plates _____

5. Very hard bone with few spaces _____

EXERCISE 6-4

Fill in the blank after each statement—does it apply to red marrow (R) or yellow marrow (Y)?

1. Found in the spaces of spongy bone _____

2. Composed largely of fat _____

3. Site of blood cell synthesis _____

4. Found in the shaft of a long bone _____

EXERCISE 6-5

Write the appropriate term in each blank from the list below.

diaphysis   epiphysis   medullary cavity   central canal
periosteum   endosteum   spongy bone   osteon

1. The shaft of a long bone   _____

2. The tough connective tissue membrane that covers bones   _____

3. The end of a long bone   _____

4. The type of bone tissue found at the end of long bones   _____

5. The thin membrane that lines the central cavity of long bones   _____

6. The hollow portion of a long bone containing yellow marrow   _____

7. The longitudinal canal in the middle of each osteon   _____

4. NAME THE THREE DIFFERENT TYPES OF CELLS IN BONE AND DESCRIBE THE FUNCTIONS OF EACH.

EXERCISE 6-6

Write the name of the appropriate bone cell in each blank from the list below.

osteoblast   osteocyte   osteoclast

1. A cell that resorbs bone matrix   _____

2. A mature bone cell that is completely surrounded by
   hard bone tissue   _____

3. A cell that builds bone tissue   _____

5. EXPLAIN HOW A LONG BONE GROWS.

EXERCISE 6-7

Label each of the following statements as true (T) or false (F).

1. Long bones grow in length by producing new bone tissue
   in the middle of the diaphysis.   _____

2. Once bone growth is complete, the epiphyseal plate turns
   into the epiphyseal line.   _____

3. Long bones elongate by converting cartilage in the bone ends
   into bone tissue.   _____

4. Osteoclasts and osteoblasts stop working once bone growth
   is complete.   _____

5. As a bone lengthens, the medullary cavity becomes larger.   _____

6. NAME AND DESCRIBE VARIOUS MARKINGS FOUND ON BONES.

EXERCISE 6-8

Write the appropriate term in each blank below and on the next page from the list below.

crest   condyle   head   process
foramen   fossa   sinus   meatus

1. A short channel or passageway   _____

2. An air space found in some skull bones   _____

3. A rounded knoblike end separated by a slender region
   from the rest of the bone   _____

4. A rounded projection   _____

5. A distinct border or ridge   _____

6. A depression on a bone surface   _____

7. A hole that permits the passage of a vessel or nerve   _____

7. NAME, LOCATE, AND DESCRIBE THE BONES IN THE AXIAL SKELETON.

EXERCISE 6-9: The Skull (Text Fig. 6-5)

1. Color the boxes next to the names of the skull bones in different, light colors.

2. Color the skull bones with the corresponding color.

3. Label each of the following numbered bones and bone features (write their names in black).

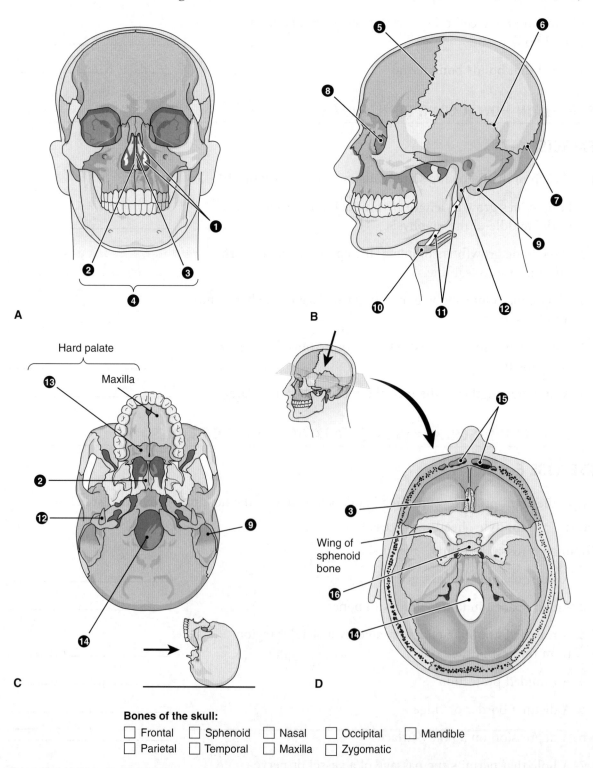

Bones of the skull:

☐ Frontal   ☐ Sphenoid   ☐ Nasal   ☐ Occipital   ☐ Mandible
☐ Parietal   ☐ Temporal   ☐ Maxilla   ☐ Zygomatic

1. _____

2. _____

3. _____

4. _____

5. _____

6. _____

7. _____

8. _____

9. _____

10. _____

11. _____

12. _____

13. _____

14. _____

15. _____

16. _____

EXERCISE 6-10: The Skull: Sagittal Section (Text Fig. 6-6)

1. Use the same colors you used in Exercise 6-9 to color bones 2, 3, 9, 10, 11, and 12. Write the name of the bone on the corresponding line in the same color.
2. Write the name of all other bones and features in black on the corresponding line.

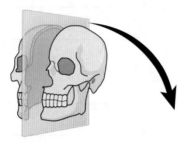

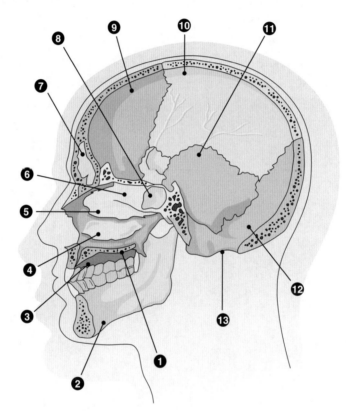

1. _____   8. _____

2. _____   9. _____

3. _____   10. _____

4. _____   11. _____

5. _____   12. _____

6. _____   13. _____

7. _____

EXERCISE 6-11: Bones of the Thorax, Anterior View (Text Fig. 6-11)

1. Write the name of each labeled part on the lines beside the bullets in different colors.
   Structures 1, 3, 6, 7 will not be colored, so write their names in black.
2. Color the different structures on the diagram with the corresponding color.

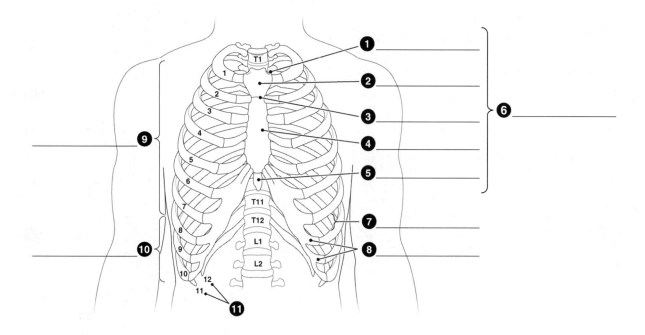

EXERCISE 6-12: Vertebral Column, Left Lateral View (Text Fig. 6-8)

1. Color each of the following bones the indicated color.
    a. cervical vertebrae—blue
    b. thoracic vertebrae—red
    c. lumbar vertebrae—green
    d. sacrum—yellow
    e. coccyx—violet
2. Label each of the indicated bones and bone parts.

1. _____

2. _____

3. _____

4. _____

5. _____

6. _____

7. _____

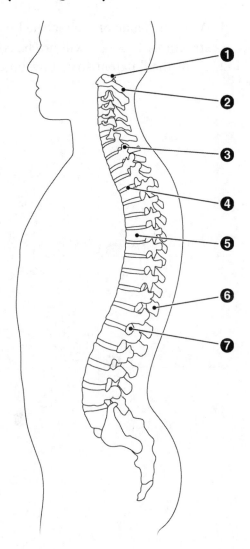

EXERCISE 6-13: The Vertebral Column and Vertebrae (Text Fig. 6-9)

1. Write the names of the three vertebral divisions in the numbered boxes 1 to 3.
2. Write the name of each labeled part on the numbered lines in different colors.
3. Color the different structures on the diagram with the corresponding color.

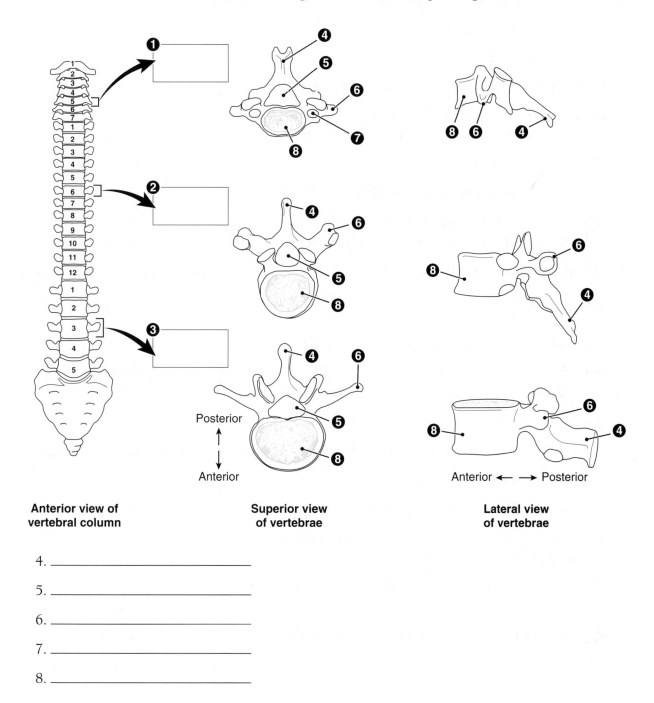

Anterior view of
vertebral column

Superior view
of vertebrae

Lateral view
of vertebrae

4. _____

5. _____

6. _____

7. _____

8. _____

EXERCISE 6-14

Write the appropriate term in each blank from the list below.

parietal bone   temporal bone   frontal bone   hyoid bone   nasal bone   occipital bone
maxilla   mandible   sphenoid bone   zygomatic bone

1. The only movable bone of the skull   _____

2. A bone of the upper jaw   _____

3. The U-shaped bone lying just below the mandible   _____

4. The bone that articulates with the parietal and temporal
   bones and forms the posterior inferior part of the cranium   _____

5. The bone that forms the forehead   _____

6. One of two slender bones that form the bridge of the nose   _____

7. One of two large bones that articulate with the frontal bone
   and form the superior lateral portions of the cranium   _____

8. The anatomic name for the cheekbone   _____

EXERCISE 6-15

Write the appropriate term in each blank from the list below.

floating ribs   true ribs   fontanel   costal   foramina
xiphoid process   manubrium   clavicular notch

1. The T-shaped, superior portion of the sternum   _____

2. The portion of the sternum that is made of cartilage in children _____

3. An adjective that refers to the ribs   _____

4. A soft spot in the infant skull that later closes   _____

5. The last two pairs of ribs, which are very short and do not
   extend to the front of the body   _____

6. The point of articulation between the sternum and the
   collarbone   _____

7. Ribs that attach to the sternum by individual cartilages   _____

8. DESCRIBE THE NORMAL CURVES OF THE SPINE AND EXPLAIN THEIR PURPOSE.

EXERCISE 6-16

Write the appropriate term in each blank from the list below.

cervical region   thoracic region   lumbar region   coccyx

thoracic curve   lumbar curve   cervical curve

1. A primary curve of the spine _____

2. The second part of the vertebral column, made up of 12 vertebrae _____

3. The spinal curve that appears when the infant holds his or her head up _____

4. The spinal curve that appears when the infant begins to walk _____

5. The most inferior part of the vertebral column _____

6. The region of the spine that contains the largest, strongest vertebrae _____

7. The region of the vertebral column made up of the first seven vertebrae _____

9. NAME, LOCATE, AND DESCRIBE THE BONES IN THE APPENDICULAR SKELETON.

EXERCISE 6-17: The Skeleton (Text Fig. 6-1)

1. Write the name of each labeled part on the lines beside the bullets in different colors. Use the same color for structures 23 to 25 and for structures 19 and 20.
2. Color the different structures on the diagram with the corresponding color. Try to color every structure in the figure with the appropriate color. For instance, structure number 3 is found in two locations.

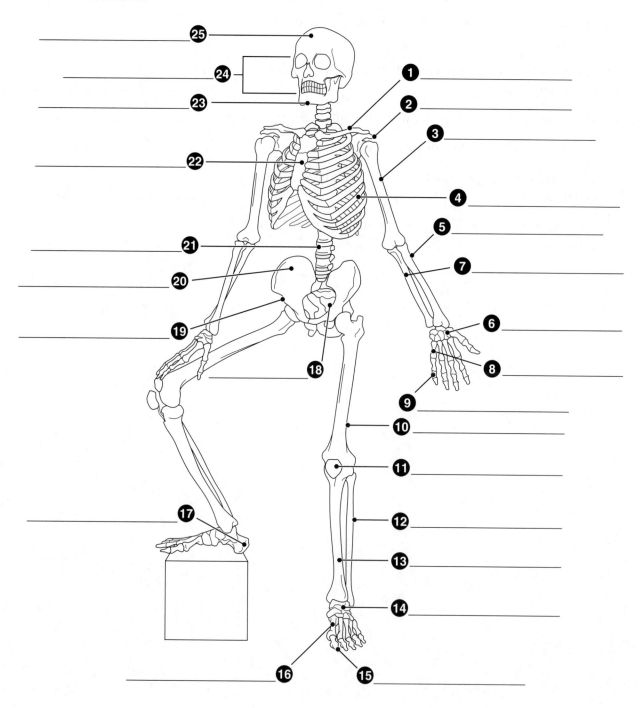

EXERCISE 6-18: The Shoulder Girdle (Text Fig. 6-12)

1. Use three contrasting colors to write the names of the illustrated bones in lines 1, 4, and 5. Color the bones the corresponding colors.
2. Write the names of the bone features in black on the other numbered lines.

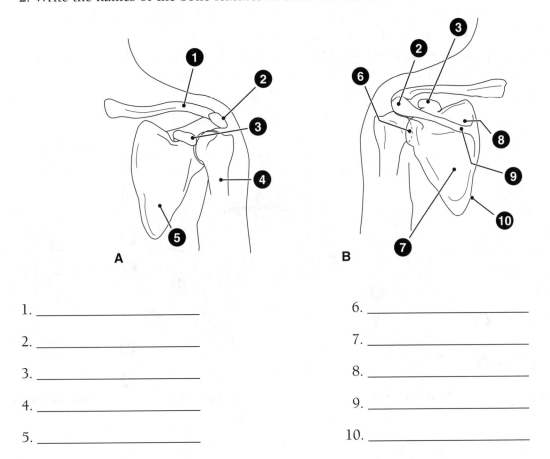

A

B

1. _____

2. _____

3. _____

4. _____

5. _____

6. _____

7. _____

8. _____

9. _____

10. _____

EXERCISE 6-19: Bones of the Upper Extremity (Text Fig. 6-13)

1. Color the large bone in part A with a bright color. Use this color to write the name of the bone in the first line, and all of its features on lines 2 to 6.
2. Write the name of the joint indicated by bullet 7 on line 7.
3. Use a bright color to shade and write the name of the bone indicated by bullet 8. Use the same color to write the name of this bone's features (bullets 9–10).
4. Use a contrasting color to shade and write the name of the bone indicated by bullet 11. Use the same color to write the name of this bone's features (bullets 12–16).

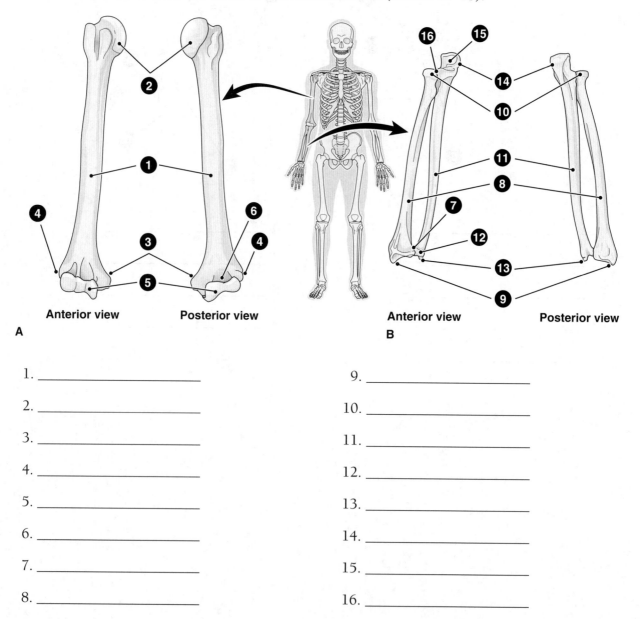

Anterior view   Posterior view   Anterior view   Posterior view

A   B

1. _____   9. _____

2. _____   10. _____

3. _____   11. _____

4. _____   12. _____

5. _____   13. _____

6. _____   14. _____

7. _____   15. _____

8. _____   16. _____

EXERCISE 6-20: Pelvic Bones (Text Fig. 6-17)

1. Color the boxes next to the names of the pelvic bones in different, light colors.
2. Color the pelvic bones in parts A and B of the diagram with the corresponding color.
3. Label each of the following numbered bones and bone features.

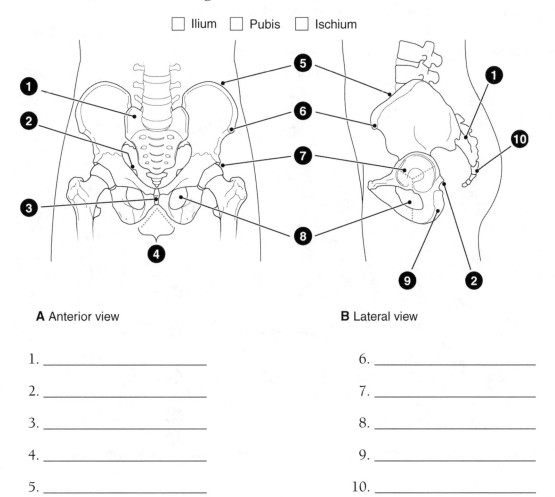

☐ Ilium   ☐ Pubis   ☐ Ischium

A Anterior view   **B** Lateral view

1. _____   6. _____

2. _____   7. _____

3. _____   8. _____

4. _____   9. _____

5. _____   10. _____

EXERCISE 6-21: Bones of the Lower Extremity (Text Fig. 6-19)

1. Color the large bone in part A with a bright color. Use this color to write the name of the bone in the first line, and all of its features on lines 2 to 10.
2. Use a bright color to shade and write the name of the bone indicated by bullet 11. Use the same color to write the name of this bone's features (bullets 12–16).
3. Use a contrasting color to shade and write the name of the bone indicated by bullet 17. Use the same color to write the name of this bone's features (bullets 18–19).
4. Use black to write the name of the joints indicated by bullets 20 and 21 on the appropriate lines.

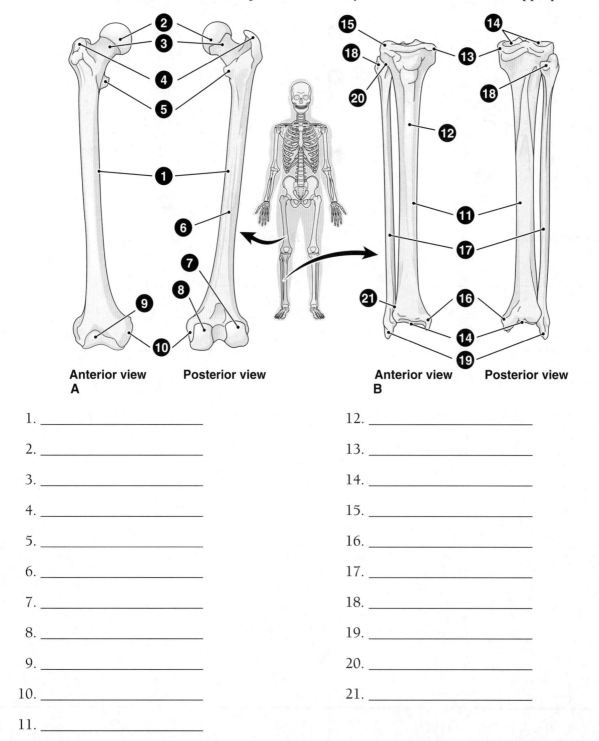

Anterior view	Posterior view	Anterior view	Posterior view
A		B	

1. _____

2. _____

3. _____

4. _____

5. _____

6. _____

7. _____

8. _____

9. _____

10. _____

11. _____

12. _____

13. _____

14. _____

15. _____

16. _____

17. _____

18. _____

19. _____

20. _____

21. _____

EXERCISE 6-22

Write the appropriate term in each blank from the list below.

olecranon   carpal bones   clavicle   ulna   radius

metacarpal bones   phalanges   scapula   humerus

1. The anatomic name for the collarbone   _____

2. The five bones in the palm of the hand   _____

3. The medial forearm bone (in the anatomic position)   _____

4. The upper part of the ulna, which forms the point of the elbow   _____

5. The 14 small bones that form the framework of the fingers
   on each hand   _____

6. The bone located on the thumb side of the forearm   _____

7. The bone containing the supraspinous and infraspinous fossae   _____

EXERCISE 6-23

Write the appropriate term in each blank from the list below.

greater trochanter   patella   tibia   calcaneus   pubis

fibula   ilium   ischium   acetabulum

1. The deep socket in the hip bone that holds the head of
   the femur   _____

2. The most inferior bone in the pelvis   _____

3. The lateral bone of the leg   _____

4. A bone that is wider and more flared in females   _____

5. The scientific name for the kneecap   _____

6. The largest of the tarsal bones; the heel bone   _____

7. The large, rounded projection at the upper and lateral
   portion of the femur   _____

EXERCISE 6-24

Write "male" or "female" in the spaces below to make each statement true.

1. The pelvic outlet is narrower in the _____ than in the _____.

2. The angle of the pubic arch is broader in the _____ than in the _____.

3. The sacrum and coccyx are shorter and less curved in the _____ than in the _____.

4. The ilia are narrower in the _____ than in the _____.

10. DESCRIBE THREE TYPES OF JOINTS AND GIVE EXAMPLES OF EACH.

EXERCISE 6-25

Write the most appropriate term in each blank. Each term will be used once.

cartilaginous joint   articulation   diarthrosis   amphiarthrosis

synarthrosis   fibrous joint   synovial joint

1. The region where two or more bones unite; a joint _____

2. A slightly moveable joint, defined by its function _____

3. A freely moveable joint, defined by its function _____

4. An immovable joint, defined by its function _____

5. A joint held together by fibrous connective tissue _____

6. A joint held together by cartilage _____

7. A joint in which there is a fluid-filled space between the bones _____

EXERCISE 6-26: The Knee Joint (Text Fig. 6-22)

1. Write the name of each labeled part on the numbered lines in different colors. Use a dark color for part 7, which can be outlined.
2. Color the different structures on the diagram with the corresponding color. Try to color every structure in the figure with the appropriate color. For instance, structure number 2 is found in two locations.

1. _____

2. _____

3. _____

4. _____

5. _____

6. _____

7. _____

8. _____

9. _____

10. _____

11. _____

12. _____

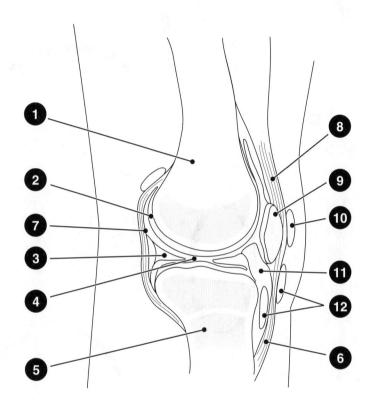

11. DEMONSTRATE SIX TYPES OF MOVEMENT THAT OCCUR AT SYNOVIAL JOINTS.

EXERCISE 6-27: Movements at Synovial Joints (Text Fig. 6-23)

Label each of the illustrated motions with the correct terms.

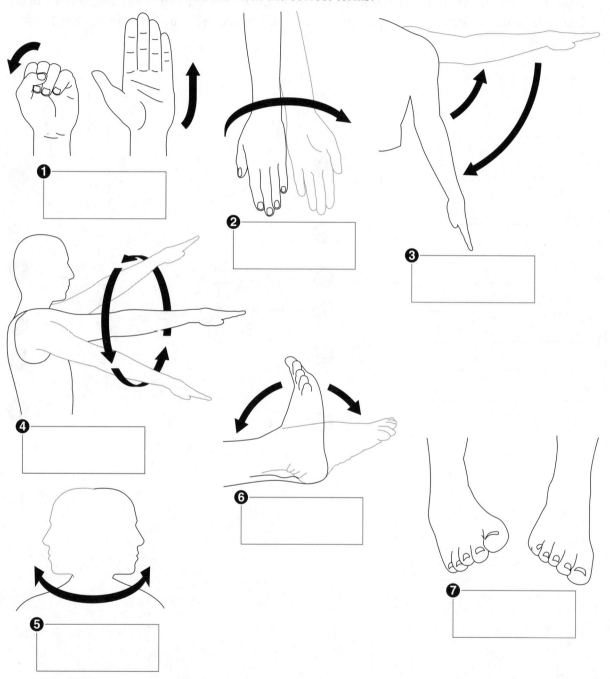

EXERCISE 6-28

Write the appropriate term in each blank from the list below.

flexion   rotation   abduction   extension   adduction
supination circumduction dorsiflexion plantar flexion pronation

1. A movement that increases the angle between two bones   _____

2. Movement away from the midline of the body   _____

3. Motion around a central axis   _____

4. A bending motion that decreases the angle between two parts   _____

5. Movement toward the midline of the body   _____

6. The act of turning the palm up or forward   _____

7. The act of pointing the toes downward   _____

EXERCISE 6-29: Types of Synovial Joints (Text Table 6-3)

Label each of the different types of synovial joints.

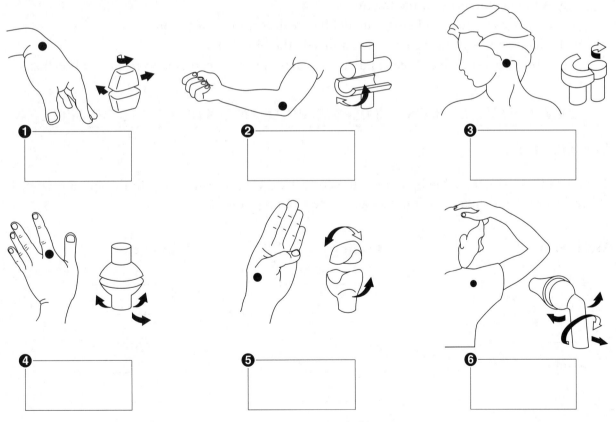

❶ _____

❷ _____

❸ _____

❹ _____

❺ _____

❻ _____

12. DESCRIBE HOW THE SKELETAL SYSTEM CHANGES WITH AGE.

EXERCISE 6-30

Write the appropriate term in each blank from the following list: protein, intervertebral discs, collagen, calcium, intercostal cartilages.

In older adults, bones are weaker because of a loss in (1) _____ salts and a general decline in the manufacture of (2) _____. Height may be reduced because the (3) _____ become thinner. The chest may become smaller because the (4) _____ become calcified and less flexible. The reduction in levels of the protein (5) _____ in tendons and ligaments makes movement more difficult.

13. USING THE CASE STUDY, DISCUSS THE PROCESS OF BONE REPAIR.

EXERCISE 6-31

The following five steps detail how Reggie's femur fracture healed, but they are out of order. Put them in order by numbering the steps 1 to 5 in the order in which they occurred.

_____ a. Osteoblasts deposit spongy bone, forming a hard callus.
_____ b. A blood clot forms at the fracture site.
_____ c. Osteoclasts and osteoblasts remodel hard callus into normal bone.
_____ d. Blood vessels from the periosteum invade the blood clot.
_____ e. Fibroblasts secrete collagen and chondrocytes produce cartilage to make a soft callus.

14. SHOW HOW WORD PARTS ARE USED TO BUILD WORDS RELATED TO THE SKELETON.

EXERCISE 6-32

Complete the following table by writing the correct word part or meaning in the space provided. Write a word that contains each word part in the Example column.

Word Part	Meaning	Example
1. pariet/o	_____	_____
2. -clast	_____	_____
3. _____	rib	_____
4. amphi-	_____	_____
5. arthr/o	_____	_____
6. _____	away from	_____
7. _____	around	_____
8. _____	toward, added to	_____
9. dia-	_____	_____

Making the Connections

The following concept map deals with bone structure. Complete the concept map by filling in the appropriate term or phrase that describes the indicated structure or process.

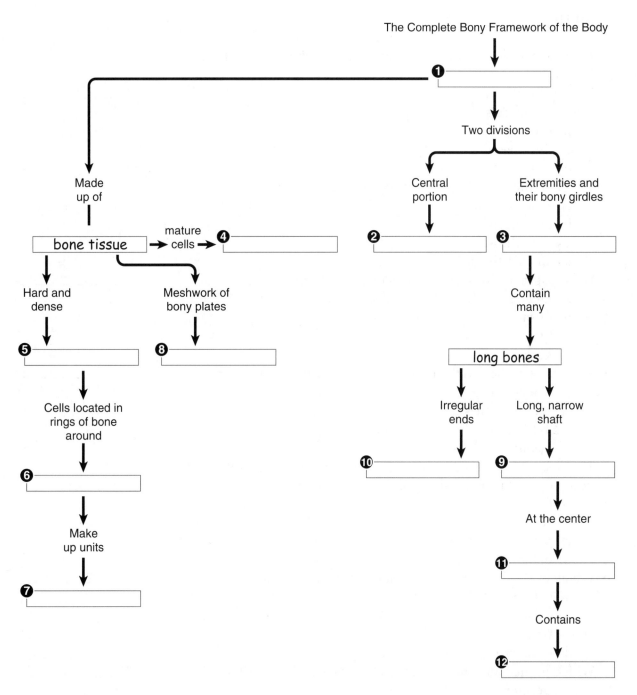

Optional Exercise: Make your own concept map, based on the different bone markings. Choose your own terms to incorporate into your map, or use the following list: bone markings, projections, depressions, head, process, condyle, crest, spine, foramen, sinus, fossa, meatus, sella turcica, mastoid sinus, foramen magnum, acromion, intervertebral foramina, supraspinous fossa, scapula spine. Try to find an example of each bone marking.

Testing Your Knowledge

BUILDING UNDERSTANDING

I. MULTIPLE CHOICE

Select the best answer and write the letter of your choice in the blank.

1. What cells dissolve bone matrix?   1. _____
   a. osteoblasts
   b. osteocytes
   c. osteoclasts
   d. osteons
2. Which of the following terms best describes sutures?   2. _____
   a. synovial joint
   b. diarthrosis
   c. synarthrosis
   d. amphiarthrosis
3. Which of the following is a projection?   3. _____
   a. process
   b. fossa
   c. foramen
   d. sinus
4. What bone makes up the posterior portion of the hard palate?   4. _____
   a. vomer bone
   b. palatine bones
   c. hyoid bone
   d. mandible
5. The os coxae is a fused bone consisting of the ilium, ischium, and a third bone. What is the name of this third bone?   5. _____
   a. femur
   b. acetabulum
   c. sacrum
   d. pubis
6. Which of the following terms best describes the patella?   6. _____
   a. sesamoid
   b. axial
   c. tarsal
   d. symphysis
7. Which of the following bones is part of the shoulder girdle?   7. _____
   a. sternum
   b. tibia
   c. scapula
   d. os coxae
8. Which rib type attaches to the sternum by individual costal cartilages?   8. _____
   a. false ribs
   b. floating ribs
   c. xiphoid ribs
   d. true ribs

9. Which of the following describes the foramen magnum?   9. _____
    a. a large hole in a hip bone near the symphysis pubis
    b. the curved rim along the top of the hip bone
    c. a hole between vertebrae that allows for passage of a spinal nerve
    d. a large opening at the base of the skull through which the spinal cord passes
10. Which of the following joint types is only capable of flexion
    and extension?   10. _____
    a. pivot
    b. ball and socket
    c. hinge
    d. gliding

II. COMPLETION EXERCISE

Write the word or phrase that correctly completes each sentence.

1. The first cervical vertebra is called the _____.

2. The bat-shaped bone that extends behind the eyes and also forms part of the base of the skull is called the _____.

3. The bone located between the eyes that extends into the nasal cavity, eye sockets, and cranial floor is called the _____.

4. The hard bone matrix is composed mainly of salts of the element _____.

5. The greater and lesser trochanters are found on the _____.

6. The small fluid-filled sacs near some joints are called _____.

7. Pivot, hinge, and gliding joints are examples of freely movable joints, also called _____.

8. Swimming the overhead crawl requires a broad circular movement at the shoulder that is a combination of simpler movements. This combined motion is called _____.

9. When you bend your foot upward to walk on your heels, the position of the foot is technically called _____.

10. In the embryo, most of the developing bones are made of _____.

11. The type of bone tissue that makes up the shaft of a long bone is called _____.

UNDERSTANDING CONCEPTS

I. TRUE/FALSE

For each question, write T for true or F for false in the blank to the left of each number. If a statement is false, correct it by replacing the underlined term and write the correct statement in the blanks below the question.

_____ 1. The shaft of a long bone contains <u>yellow</u> marrow.

_____

_____ 2. The ethmoid bone is in the <u>axial</u> skeleton.

_____

_____ 3. Moving a bone toward the midline is <u>abduction.</u>

_____

_____ 4. The pointed projection of the ulna on the posterior surface of the elbow is called the <u>axis.</u>

_____

_____ 5. Increasing the angle at a joint is <u>extension.</u>

_____

_____ 6. There are <u>six</u> pairs of false ribs.

_____

_____ 7. A mature bone cell is an <u>osteocyte.</u>

_____

_____ 8. <u>Immovable</u> joints are called synovial joints.

_____

_____ 9. The ends of a long bone are composed mainly of <u>spongy</u> bone.

_____

_____ 10. The medial malleolus is found at the distal end of the <u>fibula.</u>

_____

II. PRACTICAL APPLICATIONS

Ms M, aged 67, suffered a serious fall at a recent bowling tournament. As a physician assistant trainee, you are responsible for her preliminary evaluation.

1. Her right forearm is bent at a peculiar angle. You suspect a fracture to the radius or to the
   _____.

2. Ms M is cradling her upper extremity at the elbow. The projection of the humerus participating in the elbow joint is the _____.

3. Based on the types of movement it normally permits, the elbow joint is classified as a(n)
   _____.

4. The arm x-ray also reveals a number of fractures in the wrist bones, which are also called the
   _____.

5. Ms M also reports pain in the hip region. The hip joint consists of the femur and a deep
   socket called the _____.

6. An x-ray reveals a crack in one of the "sitting bones" that support the weight of the trunk
   when sitting. This bone is called the _____.

7. The large number of fractures Ms M suffered suggests that she may have a bone disorder. The
   physician prescribes a new medication designed to increase the activity of cells that synthesize new bone tissue. These cells are called _____.

III. SHORT ESSAYS

1. What is the function of the fontanels?

   _____

   _____

   _____

2. Describe the four curves of the adult spine and explain the purpose of these curves.

   _____

   _____

   _____

3. What is the difference between true ribs, false ribs, and floating ribs?

   _____

   _____

   _____

4. List the bones that make up the elbow joint, and describe three different articulations
   between these three bones.

   _____

   _____

   _____

CONCEPTUAL THINKING

1. The following questions relate to the knee joint.

    a. Classify the knee joint in terms of the **degree** of movement permitted.

    _____

    b. Classify the knee joint based on the **types** of movement permitted.

    _____

    c. Classify the knee joint in terms of the material between the adjoining bones.

    _____

    d. List the bones that articulate within the capsule of the knee joint.

    _____

    e. List the types of movement that can occur at the knee joint.

    _____

2. List, in order, the movements (e.g., abduction) that must occur in order to accomplish the following actions:

    a. A child brings her leg far behind her and then kicks the ball, bringing her leg in front of her.

    _____

    b. You hear your friend shouting, and turn your head to the right in the direction of the sound.

    _____

    c. The person in the car next to you bends his arm at the elbow to scratch his nose, and then straightens his arm again.

    _____

3. Using Figures 6-5 and 6-6 for reference, list all of the bones that make up the eye socket.

    _____

    _____

    _____

Expanding Your Horizons

The human skeleton has evolved from that of four-legged animals. Unfortunately, the adaptation is far from perfect; thus, our upright posture causes problems like backache and knee injuries. If you could design the human skeleton from scratch, what would you change? A *Scientific American* article suggests some improvements

• Olshansky JS, Carnes BA, Butler RN. If humans were built to last. Sci Am 2001;284:50–55.

CHAPTER 7

The Muscular System

Overview

There are three basic types of muscle tissue: skeletal, smooth, and cardiac. This chapter focuses on **skeletal muscle**, which is usually attached to bones. Skeletal muscle is also called **voluntary muscle**, because it is normally under conscious control. The muscular system is composed of more than 650 individual muscles.

Skeletal muscles are activated by electrical impulses from the nervous system. A neuron (nerve cell) makes contact with a muscle cell at the **neuromuscular junction**. The neurotransmitter **acetylcholine** transmits the signal from the neuron to the muscle cell by producing an electrical change called the **action potential** in the muscle cell membrane. The action potential causes the release of **calcium** from specialized endoplasmic reticulum (known as **sarcoplasmic reticulum**) into the muscle cell cytoplasm (known as the **sarcoplasm**). Calcium enables two types of intracellular filaments inside the muscle cell, made of **actin** and **myosin**, to contact each other. The myosin filaments pull the actin filaments closer together, resulting in muscle contraction. **ATP** is the direct source of energy for the contraction, and it is made on demand by muscle cells. Only a small amount of ATP can be synthesized without oxygen (**anaerobically**), from creatine phosphate and glucose. Most ATP is synthesized from glucose and fatty acids by **oxidation**, a process that requires adequate amounts of oxygen and mitochondria. A reserve supply of glucose is stored in muscle cells in the form of **glycogen**. Additional oxygen is stored by a muscle cell pigment called **myoglobin**.

Muscles usually work in groups to execute a body movement. The muscle that produces a given movement is called the **prime mover**; the muscle that produces the opposite action is the **antagonist**.

Muscles act with the bones of the skeleton as lever systems, in which the joint is the pivot point or fulcrum. Exercise and proper body mechanics help maintain muscle health and effectiveness. Continued activity delays the undesirable effects of aging.

This chapter contains some challenging concepts, particularly in respect to the mechanism of muscle contraction, and many muscles to memorize. Try to learn the muscle names and actions by using your own body. You should be familiar with the different movements and the anatomy of joints from Chapter 6 before you tackle this chapter.

Addressing the Learning Outcomes

1. COMPARE THE THREE TYPES OF MUSCLE TISSUE.

EXERCISE 7-1

Write the appropriate term in each blank from the list below.

cardiac muscle   skeletal muscle   tendon   fascicle   ligament

endomysium   smooth muscle   perimysium   epimysium

1. A cordlike structure that attaches a muscle to bone

   _____

2. A bundle of muscle fibers

   _____

3. A connective tissue layer surrounding muscle fiber bundles

   _____

4. Muscle under voluntary control

   _____

5. The only muscle type that does not have visible striations

   _____

6. An involuntary muscle containing intercalated disks

   _____

7. The innermost layer of the deep fascia that surrounds the entire muscle

   _____

8. The connective tissue membrane surrounding individual muscle cells

   _____

EXERCISE 7-2: Structure of a Skeletal Muscle (Text Fig. 7-1)

Label each of the indicated parts. Hint: Parts 3, 4, and 5 are membranes.

1. _____

2. _____

3. _____

4. _____

5. _____

6. _____

7. _____

8. _____

9. _____

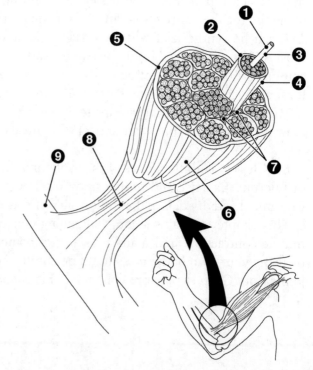

2. DESCRIBE THREE FUNCTIONS OF SKELETAL MUSCLE.

EXERCISE 7-3

List three functions of skeletal muscle in the spaces below.

1. _____

2. _____

3. _____

3. EXPLAIN HOW SKELETAL MUSCLES CONTRACT.

EXERCISE 7-4: Neuromuscular Junction (Text Fig. 7-2)

Label each of the indicated parts. Hint: Part 8 is a chemical.

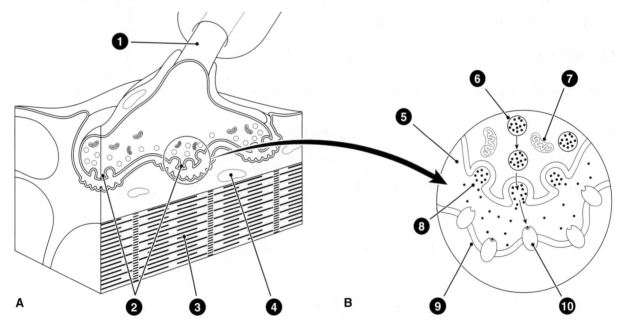

1. _____

2. _____

3. _____

4. _____

5. _____

6. _____

7. _____

8. _____

9. _____

10. _____

EXERCISE 7-5

Write the appropriate term in each blank from the list below.

synaptic cleft   motor end plate   motor unit   actin   sarcoplasmic reticulum

myosin   troponin   sarcomere   tropomyosin

1. The protein that makes up muscle's lighter, thin filaments   _____

2. The protein that interacts with actin to form crossbridges   _____

3. The membrane of the muscle cell that binds ACh   _____

4. The space between the neuron and the muscle cell   _____

5. A single neuron and all of the muscle fibers it stimulates   _____

6. A protein that binds calcium during muscle contraction   _____

7. The organelle that stores calcium in resting muscle cells   _____

8. A contracting subunit of skeletal muscle   _____

EXERCISE 7-6

In the blanks, write the name of the substance that is accomplishing each action. Each term may be used more than once.

ATP   calcium   acetylcholine

myoglobin   creatine phosphate   glycogen

1. Substance released into the synaptic cleft   _____

2. The immediate source of energy for muscle contraction   _____

3. Binds to troponin when muscle contracts   _____

4. Used to detach the myosin head   _____

5. Pumped back into the ER when muscle relaxes   _____

6. Causes an action potential when it binds the motor end plate   _____

7. A compound similar to ATP that can be used to generate ATP   _____

8. A polysaccharide that can be used to generate glucose   _____

9. A compound that stores oxygen within muscle cells   _____

EXERCISE 7-7

The events of muscle contraction are listed below, but they are out of order. Number the steps in the order in which they occur by writing the correct number in the blank. The first step has been numbered for you.

__1__ a. Acetylcholine (ACh) is released from an axon terminal into the synaptic cleft at the neuromuscular junction.

_____ b. Using stored energy, myosin heads pull actin filaments together within the sarcomeres and the cell shortens.

_____ c. Myosin heads bind to actin, forming crossbridges.

_____ d. ACh binds to receptors in the muscle's motor end plate and produces an action potential.

_____ e. New ATP is used to detach myosin heads and move them back to position for another "power stroke."

_____ f. The action potential travels to the sarcoplasmic reticulum (SR).

_____ g. Calcium shifts troponin and tropomyosin so that binding sites on actin are exposed.

_____ h. Muscle relaxes when stimulation ends and the calcium is pumped back into the sarcoplasmic reticulum.

_____ i. The sarcoplasmic reticulum releases calcium into the cytoplasm.

4. LIST COMPOUNDS STORED IN MUSCLE CELLS THAT ARE USED TO GENERATE ENERGY.

See Exercises 7-6 and 7-8.

5. EXPLAIN WHAT HAPPENS IN MUSCLE CELLS CONTRACTING ANAEROBICALLY.

EXERCISE 7-8

Circle all answers that are correct (there are two).
  In muscle cells contracting anaerobically:

a. creatine phosphate can generate ATP.
b. mitochondria break down fatty acids for energy.
c. lactic acid accumulation causes fatigue.
d. glycolysis can generate ATP by partially breaking down glucose.
e. muscle fatigue results when cells run out of ATP.

6. CITE THE EFFECTS OF EXERCISE ON MUSCLES.

EXERCISE 7-9

Label each of the following statements as true (T) or false (F).

1. Resistance exercise causes muscle hypertrophy. _____

2. Blood vessels constrict in actively contracting muscles. _____

3. Weight lifting is the most efficient way to improve endurance. _____

4. Regular exercise increases the number of capillaries in muscles. _____

5. Regular exercise decreases the number of mitochondria in muscles. _____.

7. COMPARE ISOTONIC AND ISOMETRIC CONTRACTIONS.

See Exercise 7-10.

8. EXPLAIN HOW MUSCLES WORK TOGETHER TO PRODUCE MOVEMENT.

EXERCISE 7-10

Write the appropriate term in each blank from the list below.

origin   agonist   antagonist   synergist
isotonic   isometric   insertion

1. A muscle acting as a helper to accomplish a particular movement _____

2. The muscle attachment joined to the more moveable part _____

3. The muscle attachment joined to the less moveable part _____

4. The muscle that produces a given movement _____

5. A muscle that relaxes during a given movement _____

6. A contraction in which the muscle shortens but muscle tension remains the same _____

7. A contraction in which muscle tension increases but muscle length is unchanged _____

EXERCISE 7-11: Muscle Attachment to Bones (Text Fig. 7-6)

Label each of the indicated parts.

1. _____

2. _____

3. _____

4. _____

5. _____

6. _____

7. _____

8. _____

9. COMPARE THE WORKINGS OF MUSCLES AND BONES TO LEVER SYSTEMS.

EXERCISE 7-12

For each of the following muscle actions, state which class of lever (1st, 2nd, or 3rd) is the most applicable.

1. Nodding the head _____

2. Performing a biceps curl _____

3. Standing on tiptoes _____

10. EXPLAIN HOW MUSCLES ARE NAMED.

EXERCISE 7-13

For each muscle name, write the characteristic(s) used for the name. Choose between the following six options: location, size, shape, direction of fibers, number of heads, action. The number of blanks indicates how many characteristics apply to each muscle. Note that femoris means thigh, brachii means arm, teres means long and round.

1. trapezius _____

2. quadriceps femoris _____ _____

3. rectus abdominus _____ _____

4. flexor carpii _____ _____

5. teres minor _____ _____

11. NAME SOME OF THE MAJOR MUSCLES IN EACH MUSCLE GROUP AND DESCRIBE THE LOCATION AND FUNCTION OF EACH.

EXERCISE 7-14: Superficial Muscles: Anterior View (Text Fig. 7-8)

1. Write the name of each labeled muscle on the numbered lines in different colors.
2. Color the different muscles on the diagram with the corresponding color.

1. _____

2. _____

3. _____

4. _____

5. _____

6. _____

7. _____

8. _____

9. _____

10. _____

11. _____

12. _____

13. _____

14. _____

15. _____

16. _____

17. _____

18. _____

19. _____

20. _____

21. _____

22. _____

23. _____

24. _____

25. _____

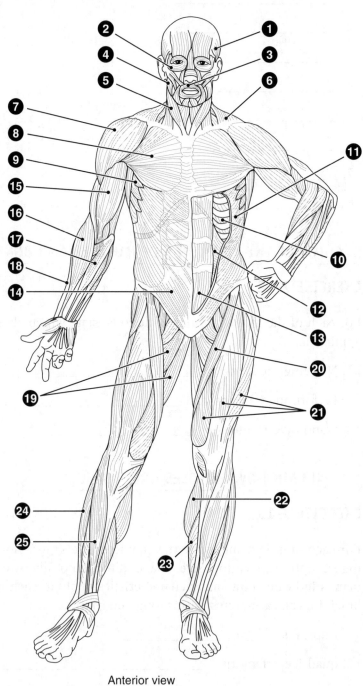

Anterior view

EXERCISE 7-15: Superficial Muscles: Posterior View (Text Fig. 7-9)

1. Write the name of each labeled muscle or tendon on the numbered lines in different colors (part 16 is a bone feature). If possible, use the same color you used for the muscle in Exercise 7-14. Note: You may need to consult Figure 7-15 in the textbook in order to label all of the muscles.

2. Color the different muscles and tendons on the diagram with the corresponding color.

1. _____
2. _____
3. _____
4. _____
5. _____
6. _____
7. _____
8. _____
9. _____
10. _____
11. _____
12. _____
13. _____
14. _____
15. _____
16. _____
17. _____
18. _____
19. _____
20. _____
21. _____

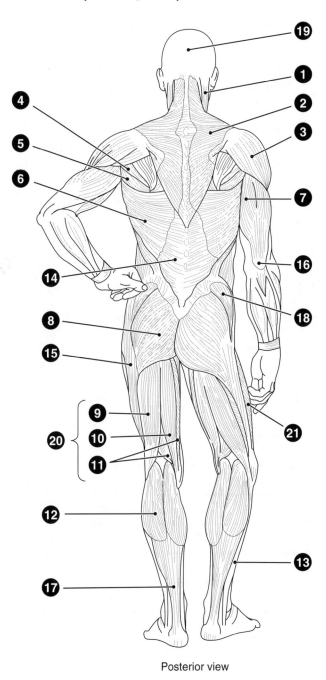

Posterior view

EXERCISE 7-16: Muscles of the Head (Text Fig. 7-10)

1. Write the name of each labeled muscle or tendon on the numbered lines in different colors. If possible, use the same color you used for the muscle in Exercises 7-14 and 7-15.
2. Color the different muscles and tendons on the diagram with the corresponding color.

1. _____

2. _____

3. _____

4. _____

5. _____

6. _____

7. _____

8. _____

9. _____

10. _____

11. _____

12. _____

13. _____

14. _____

15. _____

16. _____

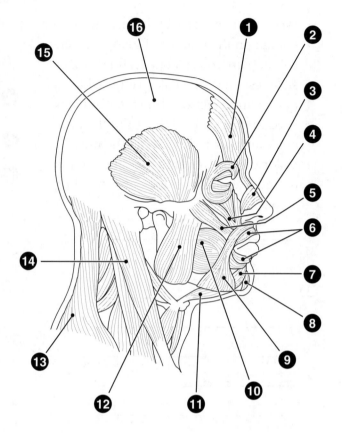

EXERCISE 7-17: Muscles of the Thigh: Anterior View (Text Fig. 7-15A)

1. Write the name of each labeled muscle, tendon or bone on the numbered lines in different colors. If possible, use the same color you used for the muscle in Exercise 7-14.
2. Color the different structures on the diagram with the corresponding color.

1. _____

2. _____

3. _____

4. _____

5. _____

6. _____

7. _____

8. _____

9. _____

10. _____

11. _____

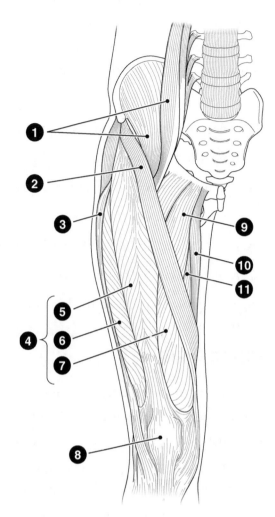

EXERCISE 7-18

Write the appropriate term in each blank from the list below.

sternocleidomastoid   buccinator   masseter   trapezius orbicularis oris

deltoid   rotator cuff   orbicularis oculi   brachialis

1. The muscle capping the shoulder and upper arm   _____

2. A deep muscle group that supports the shoulder joint   _____

3. A muscle that closes the eye   _____

4. The muscle that makes up the fleshy part of the cheek   _____

5. A muscle that closes the jaw   _____

6. A muscle on the side of the neck that flexes the head   _____

7. A main flexor of the forearm   _____

8. A triangular muscle on the back of the neck and the upper back
   that extends the head   _____

EXERCISE 7-19

Write the appropriate term in each blank from the list below.

triceps brachii   serratus anterior   brachioradialis   biceps brachii

intercostals   levator ani   erector spinae   latissimus dorsi

1. A large muscle of the middle and lower back that inserts in the
   humerus and extends the arm at the shoulder behind the back   _____

2. The muscle in the pelvic floor that aids in defecation   _____

3. A muscle on the front of the arm that flexes the elbow and
   supinates the hand   _____

4. The large muscle on the back of the arm that extends the elbow   _____

5. A chest muscle inferior to the axilla that moves the scapula
   forward   _____

6. A deep muscle that extends the vertebral column   _____

7. Muscles between the ribs that can enlarge the thoracic cavity   _____

EXERCISE 7-20

Write the appropriate term in each blank from the list below.

rectus abdominis   transversus abdominis   gluteus maximus   gluteus medius

iliopsoas   adductor longus   gracilis   biceps femoris   rectus femoris

1. Part of the quadriceps femoris muscle   _____

2. The muscle that forms much of the fleshy part of the buttock   _____

3. A deep muscle of the buttock that abducts the thigh   _____

4. A vertical muscle covering the anterior surface of the abdomen   _____

5. A muscle that aids in pressing the thighs together   _____

6. A muscle extending from the pubic bone to the tibia that adducts
   the thigh at the hip   _____

7. A powerful flexor of the thigh that arises from the ilium   _____

EXERCISE 7-21

Write the appropriate term in each blank from the list below.

sartorius   gastrocnemius   soleus   fibularis longus

tibialis anterior   quadriceps femoris   semimembranosus   flexor digitorum group

1. The thin muscle that travels down and across the medial
   surface of the thigh   _____

2. The chief muscle of the calf of the leg   _____

3. The muscle that inverts and dorsiflexes the foot   _____

4. Muscles that flex the toes   _____

5. The muscle that everts the foot   _____

6. A deep muscle that plantar flexes the foot at the ankle   _____

7. A group of four muscles forming the bulk of the anterior thigh   _____

12. DESCRIBE HOW MUSCLES CHANGE WITH AGE.

EXERCISE 7-22

List two changes that occur in aging muscles.

1. _____

2. _____

13. IDENTIFY AND LOCATE THE MUSCLES INVOLVED IN THE TESTS CARRIED OUT IN THE CASE STUDY.

EXERCISE 7-23

As you read in the case study, Sue was asked to perform various movements during her neurological exam. For each of the actions listed below, list the technical term for the movement and the muscle(s) that accomplish the movement.

	Movement (e.g., flexion)	Muscle(s) involved
Bend arm at the elbow		
Straighten arm at the elbow		
Stand on tiptoe		
Straighten leg at knee		

14. SHOW HOW WORD PARTS ARE USED TO BUILD WORDS RELATED TO THE MUSCULAR SYSTEM.

EXERCISE 7-24

Complete the following table by writing the correct word part or meaning in the space provided. Write a word that contains each word part in the Example column.

Word Part	Meaning	Example
1. _____	muscle	_____
2. brachi/o	_____	_____
3. _____	tone, tension	_____
4. erg/o	_____	_____
5. metr/o	_____	_____
6. _____	four	_____
7. _____	separation, dissolving	_____
8. _____	flesh	_____
9. vas/o	_____	_____
10. iso-	_____	_____

Making the Connections

The following concept map deals with substances and structures required for muscle contraction. Each pair of terms is linked together by a connecting phrase into a sentence. The sentence should be read in the direction of the arrow. Complete the concept map by filling in the appropriate term or phrase. There is one right answer for each term. However, there are many correct answers for the connecting phrases.

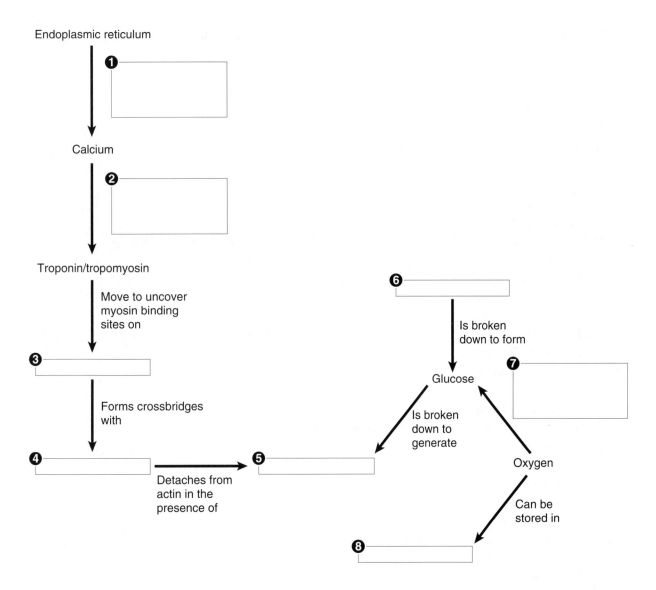

Optional Exercise: Make your own concept map, based on the events of muscle contraction. Choose your own terms to incorporate into your map, or use the following list: neuron, acetylcholine, neuromuscular junction, synaptic cleft, motor end plate, myosin, actin, endoplasmic reticulum, calcium, sarcomere, troponin/tropomyosin, ATP.

Testing Your Knowledge

BUILDING UNDERSTANDING

I. MULTIPLE CHOICE

Select the best answer and write the letter of your choice in the blank.

1. Which of the following statements is NOT true of skeletal muscle?
   a. The cells are long and threadlike.
   b. It is described as striated.
   c. It is involuntary.
   d. The cells are multinucleated.

   1. _____

2. When muscles and bones act together in the body as a lever system, what is the pivot point or fulcrum of the system?
   a. joint
   b. tendon
   c. ligament
   d. myoglobin

   2. _____

3. Which of the following is an action of the quadriceps femoris?
   a. flex the thigh
   b. extend the leg
   c. adduct the leg
   d. abduct the thigh

   3. _____

4. Which of the following is NOT a muscle of the hamstring group?
   a. biceps femoris
   b. rectus femoris
   c. semimembranosus
   d. semitendinosus

   4. _____

5. What is the name of the connective tissue layer around individual muscle fibers?
   a. epimysium
   b. perimysium
   c. superficial fascia
   d. endomysium

   5. _____

6. Where does ATP attach during muscle contraction?
   a. tropomyosin
   b. myosin
   c. actin
   d. troponin

   6. _____

7. Which of the following processes requires oxygen?
   a. ATP generation from fatty acids
   b. glycolysis
   c. creatine phosphate breakdown
   d. lactic acid synthesis

   7. _____

8. Which of these terms describes a broad tendon sheet?   8. _____
    a. ligament
    b. aponeurosis
    c. bursa
    d. meniscus

II. COMPLETION EXERCISE

Write the word or phrase that correctly completes each sentence.

1. Normally, muscles are in a partially contracted state, even when not in use. This state of mild constant tension is called _____.

2. The hemoglobin-like compound that stores oxygen in muscle is _____.

3. The muscle attachment that is usually relatively fixed is called its _____.

4. A contraction in which the muscle lengthens as it exerts force is described as _____.

5. The band of connective tissue that attaches the gastrocnemius muscle to the heel is the _____.

6. The muscles of the pelvic floor together form the _____.

7. A muscle that must relax during a given movement is called the _____.

8. The muscular partition between the thoracic and abdominal cavities is the _____.

9. A superficial muscle of the neck and upper back acts at the shoulder. This muscle is the _____.

10. The large muscle of the upper chest that flexes the arm across the body is the _____.

11. The muscle responsible for dorsiflexion and inversion of the foot is the _____.

UNDERSTANDING CONCEPTS

I. TRUE/FALSE

For each question, write T for true or F for false in the blank to the left of each number. If a statement is false, correct it by replacing the <u>underlined</u> term and write the correct statement in the blanks below the question.

_____ 1. The triceps brachii <u>flexes</u> the arm at the elbow.

_____

_____ 2. Muscle fatigue can result when <u>phosphate</u> accumulates in the cell.

_____

_____ 3. In an <u>isometric</u> contraction, muscle tension increases but the muscle does not shorten.

_____

_____ 4. A muscle that stabilizes a body part during a movement is called a(n) <u>synergist.</u>

_____

_____ 5. The neurotransmitter used at the neuromuscular junction is <u>norepinephrine.</u>

_____

_____ 6. A contracting subunit of skeletal muscle is called a(n) <u>crossbridge.</u>

_____

_____ 7. The storage form of glucose is called <u>creatine phosphate.</u>

_____

_____ 8. The element that binds to the troponin and tropomyosin complex is <u>calcium.</u>

_____

II. PRACTICAL APPLICATIONS

Study each discussion. Then, write the appropriate word or phrase in the space provided.

➤ Group A

Ms. J is sitting at her desk studying for her anatomy final exam.

1. She has excellent posture, with her back straight. The deep back muscle responsible for her erect posture is the _____.

2. Ms. J has a cheerful disposition, and she likes to whistle while she works. The cheek muscle involved in whistling is the _____.

3. Ms. J is furiously writing notes, and her hand is flexed around the pen. The muscle groups that flex the hand are called the _____.

4. After several hours of intense studying, Ms. J takes a break. Stretching, she straightens her leg at the knee joint. The muscle that accomplishes this action is the

_____.

➤ Group B

Mr. L, aged 72, is a retired concert pianist.

1. He reports numbness and weakness in his right hand. He can no longer flex and extend his fingers rapidly enough to play Rachmaninoff. The muscles that extend his fingers are the

_____.

2. Mr. L also experiences pain when he sits. He has lost muscle mass in the muscle that forms the fleshy part of the buttock, known as the _____.

3. The healthcare worker recommends that he undertakes a regular exercise program, incorporating stretching, aerobic exercise, and resistance training. Endurance training increases the quantity of a specific organelle that generates ATP aerobically. This organelle is the

_____.

4. Mr. L asks if the resistance training will give him bigger muscles. He is told that his muscle cells may increase in size, a change called _____.

III. SHORT ESSAYS

1. For each of the following word pairs, write a sentence explaining their roles in muscle contraction.
   a. glycogen and glucose

   _____

   _____

   _____

   b. calcium and oxygen

   _____

   _____

   _____

   c. acetylcholine and ATP

   _____

   _____

   _____

2. Ms. L has suffered an embarrassing (but relatively painless) fall. Mr. L is staring at her with his mouth open. Ms. L asks him to activate two muscles to close his jaw. Name these two muscles.

   _____

   _____

   _____

CONCEPTUAL THINKING

1. Your great-uncle has decided that it's time to get in shape, so he has started jogging four times weekly. He complains that he gets tired easily, because of all of the lactic acid accumulating in his muscles. Do you think he's right? Discuss the causes of muscle fatigue in your answer.

   _____

   _____

   _____

2. After 2 weeks your uncle wants to quit his exercise program, claiming that it isn't doing him any good, and makes him too tired to watch late-night hockey game reruns. What would you tell him about the benefits of endurance exercise?

_____

_____

_____

3. While attending the ballet, you notice a dancer raising her heels to stand on her tiptoes.

    a. What is the name of this action (i.e., adduction)? _____

    b. What is the agonist for this action? _____

    c. Name a synergistic muscle involved in this action. _____

    d. Name an antagonist muscle involved _____

    e. Which class of lever is represented by this action? _____

    f. Name the fulcrum and resistance, and describe the relative positions of the fulcrum, resistance, and effort.

_____

_____

_____

Expanding Your Horizons

Are world-class athletes born or made? It is no coincidence that athletic performance tends to run in families. Genetic influences on muscular function are discussed in an article in *Scientific American* (Andersen JL, Schjerling P, Saltin B. Muscle, genes and athletic performance. Sci Am 2000(September):48–55). This information could be used to screen for elite athletes—perhaps children of the future will know in which sports they can excel based on their genetic profile. This possibility is discussed in a special *Scientific American* issue entitled "Building the Elite Athlete" (Taubes G. Toward Molecular Talent Scouting. Scientific American Presents: Building the Elite Athlete 2000;11:26–31).

Coordination and Control

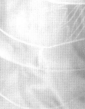

CHAPTER 8

The Nervous System: The Spinal Cord and Spinal Nerves

Overview

The nervous system is the body's coordinating system, receiving, sorting, and controlling responses to both internal and external changes (stimuli). The nervous system as a whole is divided structurally into the **central nervous system** (CNS), made up of the brain and the spinal cord, and the **peripheral nervous system** (PNS), made up of the cranial and spinal nerves. The PNS connects all parts of the body with the CNS. The brain and cranial nerves are the subject of Chapter 10. Functionally, the peripheral nervous system is divided into the somatic (voluntary) system and the autonomic (involuntary) system.

The nervous system functions by means of the **nerve impulse**, an electrical current or **action potential** that spreads along the membrane of the **neuron** (nerve cell). Each neuron is composed of a cell body and fibers, which are threadlike extensions from the cell body. A **dendrite** is a fiber that carries impulses toward the cell body, and an **axon** is a fiber that carries impulses away from the cell body. Some axons are covered with a sheath of fatty material called **myelin**, which insulates the fiber and speeds conduction along the fiber. In the PNS, neuron fibers are collected in bundles to form **nerves**. Bundles of fibers in the CNS are called **tracts**. Nerve cells make contact at a junction called a **synapse**. Here, a nerve impulse travels across a very narrow cleft between the cells by means of a chemical referred to as a **neurotransmitter**. Neurotransmitters are released from axons of presynaptic cells to be picked up by receptors in the membranes of responding cells, the postsynaptic cells.

A neuron may be classified as a sensory (afferent) type, which carries impulses toward the CNS, or a motor (efferent) type, which carries impulses away from the CNS. **Interneurons** are connecting neurons within the CNS.

The basic functional pathway of the nervous system is the **reflex arc**, in which an impulse travels from a receptor, along a sensory neuron to a synapse or synapses in the CNS, and then along a motor neuron to an effector organ that carries out a response.

The spinal cord carries impulses to and from the brain. It is also a center for simple reflex activities in which responses are coordinated within the cord.

The **autonomic nervous system** controls unconscious activities. This system regulates the actions of glands, smooth muscle, and the heart muscle. The autonomic nervous system has two divisions, the **sympathetic nervous system** and the **parasympathetic nervous system**, which generally have opposite effects on a given organ.

Addressing the Learning Outcomes

1. OUTLINE THE ORGANIZATION OF THE NERVOUS SYSTEM ACCORDING TO STRUCTURE AND FUNCTION.

EXERCISE 8-1: Anatomic Divisions of the Nervous System (Text Fig. 8-1)

Label the parts and divisions of the nervous system shown below.

1. _____

2. _____

3. _____

4. _____

5. _____

6. _____

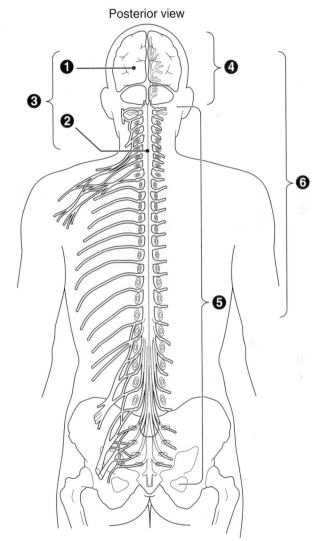

Posterior view

EXERCISE 8-2

Write the appropriate term in each blank from the list below.

central nervous system   peripheral nervous system   somatic nervous system

sympathetic nervous system   parasympathetic nervous system   autonomic nervous system

1. The functional division that controls the heart   _____

2. The functional division that controls skeletal muscles   _____

3. The system that promotes the fight-or-flight response   _____

4. The system that stimulates the activity of the digestive tract   _____

5. The structural division that includes the brain   _____

6. The structural division that includes the cranial nerves   _____

2. DESCRIBE THE STRUCTURE OF A NEURON.

EXERCISE 8-3: The Motor Neuron (Text Fig. 8-2)

1. Write the name of each labeled part on the numbered lines in different colors. Structures 4 and 5 will not be colored, so write their names in black. Use related colors for structures 4 and 6.
2. Color the different structures on the diagram with the corresponding color.
3. Add large arrows showing the direction the nerve impulse will travel from the dendrites to the muscle.

1. _____

2. _____

3. _____

4. _____

5. _____

6. _____

7. _____

8. _____

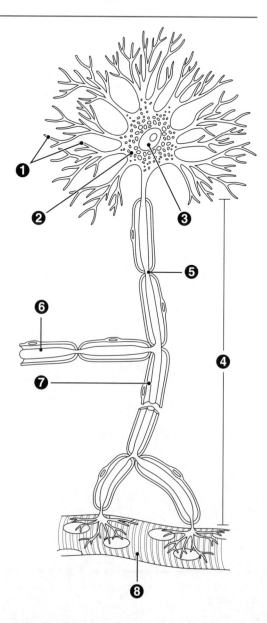

EXERCISE 8-4

Write the appropriate term in each blank from the list below.

dendrite	neurilemma	axon	Schwann cell
node	white matter	gray matter	

1. A neuron fiber that carries impulses away from the cell body _____

2. The part of a neuron that receives a stimulus _____

3. The sheath around some neuron fibers that aids in regeneration _____

4. A gap in the neuron sheath _____

5. The portion of the spinal cord made up of myelinated axons _____

6. Neural tissue composed of cell bodies and unmyelinated axons _____

3. DESCRIBE HOW NEURON FIBERS ARE BUILT INTO A NERVE.

EXERCISE 8-5

Write the appropriate term in each blank from the list below.

sensory neurons	motor neurons	neuron	tract
endoneurium	perineurium	epineurium	nerve

1. The scientific name for a nerve cell _____

2. A bundle of neuron fibers located outside the central nervous system _____

3. A bundle of neuron fibers located within the central nervous system _____

4. Neurons that conduct impulses towards the brain _____

5. Neurons that conduct impulses away from the brain _____

6. The coating of an individual neuron _____

7. The coating of an entire nerve _____

4. EXPLAIN THE PURPOSE OF NEUROGLIA.

EXERCISE 8-6

List five functions of neuroglia in the spaces below.

1. _____

2. _____

3. _____

4. _____

5. _____

5. DIAGRAM AND DESCRIBE THE STEPS IN AN ACTION POTENTIAL.

EXERCISE 8-7

In the space below, draw an action potential tracing as illustrated in Figure 8-7. On your diagram, indicate which event is occurring (depolarization, repolarization, or resting) and which ion is moving (sodium [Na^+] or potassium [K^+]), if any.

EXERCISE 8-8

Write the appropriate term in each blank from the list below.

depolarization	action potential	repolarization
resting	Na^+	K^+

1. The step in which the membrane potential returns to rest _____

2. The ion that crosses the neuron membrane to cause depolarization _____

3. The result of positive ions entering the neuron _____

4. A sudden change in membrane potential that is transmitted along axons _____

5. The ion that leaves the neuron to cause repolarization _____

6. EXPLAIN THE ROLE OF MYELIN IN NERVE CONDUCTION.

EXERCISE 8-9

Place the following events in the order in which they occur.
   a. The action potential opens sodium channels in adjacent portions of the membrane.
   b. Sodium entry into the cell causes another action potential in the adjacent portion of the membrane.
   c. A stimulus initiates an action potential.
   d. Open sodium channels let sodium enter the cell.

1. _____

2. _____

3. _____

4. _____

EXERCISE 8-10: Formation of a Myelin Sheath (Text Fig. 8-4)

1. Write the name of each labeled part on the numbered lines in different colors. Structures 5, 7, 8, and 9 will not be colored, so write their names in black.
2. Color the different structures on the diagram with the corresponding color. Make sure you color the structure in all parts of the diagram. For instance, structure 3 is visible in three locations.

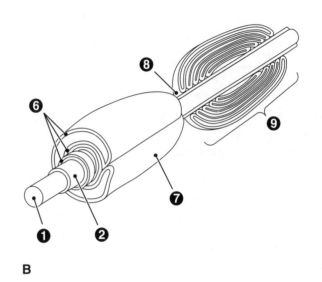

1. _____

2. _____

3. _____

4. _____

5. _____

6. _____

7. _____

8. _____

9. _____

EXERCISE 8-11

Label each of the following statements as true (T) or false (F).

1. Action potentials occur in axon regions surrounded by myelin _____

2. Action potential transmission is faster in myelinated neurons _____

3. Action potentials occur at nodes in myelinated axons _____

7. EXPLAIN THE ROLE OF NEUROTRANSMITTERS IN IMPULSE TRANSMISSION AT A SYNAPSE.

EXERCISE 8-12: A Synapse (Text Fig. 8-10)

Label the parts of the synapse shown below.

1. _____

2. _____

3. _____

4. _____

5. _____

6. _____

7. _____

8. _____

9. _____

10. _____

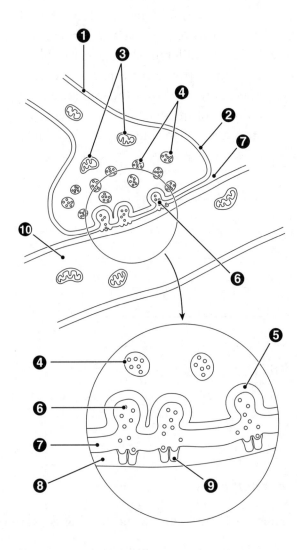

EXERCISE 8-13

Place the following events in order.

a. Neurotransmitter molecules bind to receptors in the postsynaptic membrane.
b. Neurotransmitter molecules are released into the synaptic cleft.
c. The nerve impulse arrives at the end of the presynaptic neuron.
d. Vesicles containing neurotransmitter fuse with the axonal plasma membrane.
e. The activity of the postsynaptic cell is altered.

1. _____

2. _____

3. _____

4. _____

5. _____

EXERCISE 8-14

List three examples of neurotransmitters in the spaces below.

1. _____

2. _____

3. _____

8. DESCRIBE THE DISTRIBUTION OF GRAY AND WHITE MATTER IN THE SPINAL CORD.

EXERCISE 8-15: Spinal Cord (Text Fig. 8-11B)

1. Write the name of each labeled part on the numbered lines. Use the following color scheme:
   - 1 and 2: red
   - 3, 4, 9: different dark colors
   - 5: pink
   - 6: any light color
   - 7: light blue
   - 10: medium blue
   - 11: purple
2. Color or outline the different structures on the diagram with the corresponding color.
   Color each structure on both sides of the spinal cord, not just on the side that is labeled.

1. _____   7. _____

2. _____   8. _____

3. _____   9. _____

4. _____   10. _____

5. _____   11. _____

6. _____

9. DESCRIBE AND NAME THE SPINAL NERVES AND THREE OF THEIR MAIN PLEXUSES.

EXERCISE 8-16: Spinal Cord (Text Fig. 8-11A)

Write the name of each structure on the appropriate line.

1. _____
2. _____
3. _____
4. _____
5. _____
6. _____
7. _____
8. _____
9. _____
10. _____
11. _____

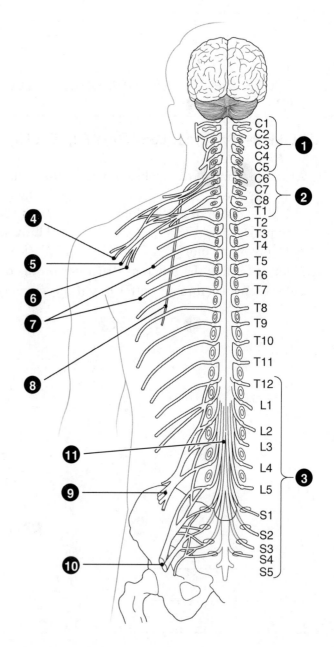

10. LIST THE COMPONENTS OF A REFLEX ARC.

EXERCISE 8-17: Reflex Arc (Text Fig. 8-13)

1. Write the names of the five components of a reflex arc on the numbered lines 1 to 5 in different colors, and color the components with the appropriate color. Follow the color scheme provided below.

2. Write the names of the parts of the spinal cord on numbered lines 6 to 12 in different colors, and color the structures with the appropriate color. Follow the color scheme provided below.

Color Scheme
- 1, 2, 6, 7, 8: red
- 3: green
- 4, 10: medium blue
- 5: purple
- 9: do not color (write name in black)
- 11: pink
- 12: light blue

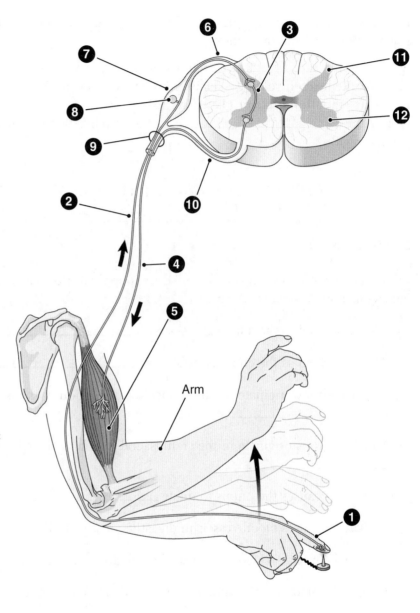

1. _____

2. _____

3. _____

4. _____

5. _____

6. _____

7. _____

8. _____

9. _____

10. _____

11. _____

12. _____

11. DEFINE A SIMPLE REFLEX AND GIVE SEVERAL EXAMPLES OF REFLEXES.

EXERCISE 8-18

Fill in the blanks in the discussion below using the following terms: patellar reflex, simple reflex, somatic reflex, autonomic reflex.

A (1) _____ reflex describes any rapid automatic response involving very few neurons. Reflexes involving skeletal muscles are called (2) _____; reflexes involving smooth muscle or glands are (3) _____. An example of the former type is the (4) _____, a stretch reflex that involves striking a tendon in the patellar region.

12. COMPARE THE LOCATION AND FUNCTIONS OF THE SYMPATHETIC AND PARASYMPATHETIC NERVOUS SYSTEMS.

EXERCISE 8-19

Fill in the blank after each statement—does it apply to the sympathetic nervous system (S) or the parasympathetic nervous system (P)?

1. Also described as the adrenergic system _____

2. Also described as the cholinergic system _____

3. Motor neurons originate in the thoracolumbar region of the spinal cord

   _____

4. Motor neurons originate in the craniosacral region of the spinal cord

   _____

5. Activation causes the pupils to dilate _____

6. Activation causes blood vessels in digestive organs to dilate _____

7. Terminal ganglia located in or near the effector _____

8. Ganglia located near the spinal cord or in collateral ganglia _____

9. Activation decreases kidney activity _____

10. Activation stimulates the sweat glands _____

13. EXPLAIN THE ROLE OF CELLULAR RECEPTORS IN THE ACTION OF NEUROTRANSMITTERS IN THE AUTONOMIC NERVOUS SYSTEM.

EXERCISE 8-20

Write the appropriate term in each blank from the list below.
muscarinic receptor   nicotinic receptor   adrenergic receptor

1. Binds norepinephrine   _____

2. Binds acetylcholine and induces muscle contraction   _____

3. Acetylcholine receptor found on effector organs of the
   parasympathetic system   _____

14. USING THE CASE STUDY, DESCRIBE THE IMPORTANCE OF MYELIN FOR NORMAL MOTOR AND SENSORY FUNCTION.

EXERCISE 8-21

Fill in the blanks in the discussion below, using the following terms (not all terms will be used); sensory, motor, descending, ascending, dorsal, ventral, myelin, multiple sclerosis, white matter, gray matter.

Sue suffered from (1) _____, a disease associated with demyelination. The (2) _____ coating of neuronal axons was destroyed by an autoimmune reaction. Lesions were apparent in the type of spinal cord tissue containing myelinated axons, known as (3) _____. Sue's sense of touch was impaired because of damage to neurons in the (4) _____ tracts of her spinal cord. These neurons are known as (5) _____, or afferent, neurons, and they receive input from neurons entering the spinal cord through the (6) _____ root. Sue's muscle control was impaired because of damage to (7) _____ neurons in the (8) _____ tracts of her spinal cord. Motor impulses from this pathway leave the spinal cord through the (9) _____ root.

15. SHOW HOW WORD PARTS ARE USED TO BUILD WORDS RELATED TO THE NERVOUS SYSTEM.

EXERCISE 8-22

Complete the following table by writing the correct word part or meaning in the space provided. Write a word that contains each word part in the "Example" column.

Word Part	Meaning	Example
1. _____	sheath	_____
2. re	_____	_____
3. soma-	_____	_____
4. _____	nerve, nervous tissue	_____
5. _____	remove	_____
6. aut/o	_____	_____
7. post-	_____	_____

Making the Connections

The following concept map deals with the organization of the nervous system. Each pair of terms is linked together by a connecting phrase into a sentence. The sentence should be read in the direction of the arrow. Complete the concept map by filling in the appropriate term or phrase. There is one right answer for each term. However, there are many correct answers for the connecting phrases (6, 7).

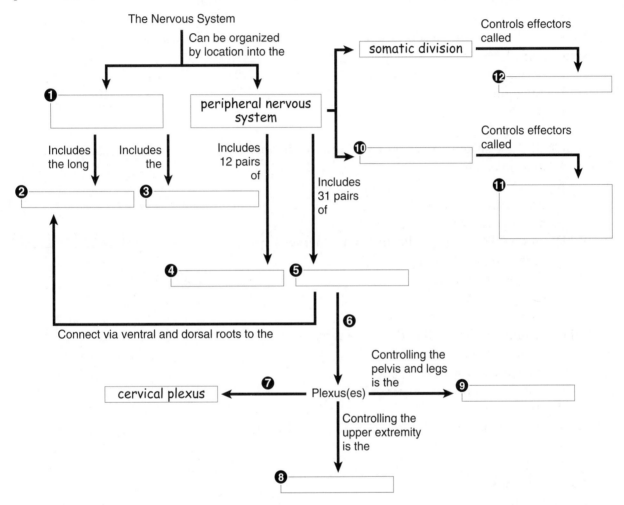

Optional Exercise: Make your own concept map, based on the structures of the spinal cord and the components of a reflex loop. Choose your own terms to incorporate into your map, or use the following list: dorsal root ganglion, gray matter, white matter, ventral root ganglion, sensory neuron, motor neuron, receptor, muscle, gland, effector.

Testing Your Knowledge

BUILDING UNDERSTANDING

I. MULTIPLE CHOICE

Select the best answer and write the letter of your choice in the blank.

1. Which of the following terms describes a skin region supplied by a single spinal nerve?
   1. _____
   a. dermatome
   b. ganglion
   c. plexus
   d. synapse

2. Which of these structures would you find in white matter?
   2. _____
   a. neuron cell bodies
   b. dendrites
   c. unmyelinated axons
   d. myelinated axons

3. Which of the following are effectors of the nervous system?
   3. _____
   a. sensory neurons and ganglia
   b. muscles and glands
   c. synapses and dendrites
   d. receptors and neurotransmitters

4. Where would you find cell bodies of sensory neurons?
   4. _____
   a. dorsal root of the spinal cord
   b. sympathetic chain
   c. ventral root of the spinal cord
   d. effector organ

5. Which of the following substances is a neurotransmitter?
   5. _____
   a. myelin
   b. actin
   c. epinephrine
   d. sebum

6. Which of these is an effector of the voluntary nervous system?
   6. _____
   a. cardiac muscle
   b. skeletal muscle
   c. smooth muscle
   d. glands

7. Which neuron type conveys impulses *within* the spinal cord?
   7. _____
   a. sensory neurons
   b. motor neurons
   c. interneurons
   d. mixed nerves

II. COMPLETION EXERCISE

Write the word or phrase that correctly completes each sentence.

1. Fibers that carry impulses toward the neuron cell body are called _____.

2. The portion of the spinal cord made up of cell bodies and unmyelinated axons is called the _____.

3. The fatty material that covers some axons is called _____.

4. Dilation of the bronchial tubes is increased by the part of the autonomic nervous system called the _____.

5. The tiny space separating the presynaptic and postsynaptic neurons is the _____.

6. The network of spinal nerves that supplies the pelvis and legs is the _____.

7. The brain and spinal cord together are referred to as the _____.

8. The neurotransmitter used at cholinergic synapses is _____.

9. The small channel in the center of the spinal cord that contains cerebrospinal fluid is the _____.

10. The ion responsible for the depolarizing phase of the action potential is _____.

11. The bridge of gray matter connecting the right and left horns of the spinal cord is the _____.

UNDERSTANDING CONCEPTS

I. TRUE/FALSE

For each question, write T for true or F for false in the blank to the left of each number. If a statement is false, correct it by replacing the underlined term and write the correct statement in the blanks below the question.

_____ 1. Motor impulses leave the dorsal horn of the spinal cord.

_____

_____ 2. An axon conducts impulses toward the cell body.

_____

_____ 3. A tract is a bundle of neuron fibers within the central nervous system.

_____

_____ 4. The <u>parasympathetic</u> system has terminal ganglia.

_____

_____ 5. The <u>brachial plexus</u> controls the shoulder and arm.

_____

_____ 6. The parasympathetic system is <u>adrenergic</u>.

_____

_____ 7. The cranial nerves are part of the <u>central</u> nervous system.

_____

_____ 8. Neurotransmitters bind to specific proteins on the postsynaptic cell called <u>transporters</u>.

_____

_____ 9. At a synapse, a neurotransmitter is released from the <u>postsynaptic</u> cell.

_____

_____ 10. A reflex arc that passes through the spinal cord but not the brain is called a <u>spinal</u> reflex.

_____

II. PRACTICAL APPLICATIONS

Study each discussion. Then write the appropriate word or phrase in the space provided.

1. Mr. W, a patient with diabetes mellitus for 10 years, complained of pain and numbness of his feet. In observing Mr. W walk, the physician noted there was weakness in the muscles responsible for dorsiflexion of the foot. The nerves that supply the foot are found in a plexus called the _____.

2. The physician pricked Mr. W's foot with a needle. Mr. W did not feel the needle prick, suggesting that there was a problem with the nerves that carry impulses to the brain. These nerves are called _____.

3. The physician tapped below Mr. W's knee to elicit a knee-jerk response. The tendon she struck was the _____.

4. When the tendon was stretched, it activated a receptor. The type of neuron that conveyed the signal from the receptor to the spinal cord is a(n) _____.

5. Mr. W knew that his tendon had been tapped, because signals passed to his brain through a nerve tract in the spinal cord called the _____.

6. The effector in this reflex arc is the _____.

III. SHORT ESSAYS

1. List the events that occur in an action potential.

_____

_____

_____

2. What are neuroglia, and what are some functions of neuroglia?

_____

_____

_____

CONCEPTUAL THINKING

1. Ms. J is teaching English in Japan. She dines on a local delicacy called pufferfish, and shortly thereafter her lips go numb. She later discovers that pufferfish contain a toxin that blocks sodium channels. Explain why her lips are numb.

_____

_____

_____

2. Dopamine is a neurotransmitter involved in feelings of pleasure. Cocaine blocks the reuptake of dopamine. Use this information to discuss how cocaine affects mood.

_____

_____

_____

Expanding Your Horizons

Christopher Reeve of *Superman* fame is probably the best known victim of a spinal cord injury. An equestrian injury pulverized his first and second cervical vertebrae, resulting in complete paralysis of his limbs and semiparalysis of his respiratory muscles. He became a strong advocate for spinal cord research, establishing the *Christopher Reeve Foundation* (now the *Christopher and Dana Reeve Foundation*) for spinal cord research and patient support. Check out the Foundation's Web site for patient stories and breaking research news, or read the article listed below about recent advances.

- Griffith A. Healing broken nerves. Sci Am 2007(September);297:28–30.
- Christopher and Dana Reeve Foundation. Available at: http://www.christopherreeve.org

CHAPTER 9

The Nervous System: The Brain and Cranial Nerves

Overview

The brain consists of the two cerebral hemispheres, the diencephalon, the brainstem, and the cerebellum. Each cerebral hemisphere is covered by a layer of gray matter, the **cerebral cortex**, which is further divided into four lobes (the frontal, parietal, temporal, and occipital lobes). Specific functions have been localized to the different lobes. For instance, the interpretation of visual images is performed by an area of the occipital lobe. The diencephalon consists of the **thalamus**, an important relay station for sensory impulses, and the **hypothalamus**, which plays an important role in homeostasis. The brainstem links the spinal cord to the brain and regulates many involuntary functions necessary for life, whereas the cerebellum is involved in coordination and balance. The **limbic system** is not found in a specific brain division. It consists of several structures located between the cerebrum and diencephalon that are involved in emotion, learning, and memory.

The brain and spinal cord are covered by three layers of fibrous membranes called the **meninges**. The **cerebrospinal fluid** (CSF) also protects the brain and spinal cord by providing support and cushioning. The CSF is produced by the choroid plexuses (capillary networks) in four ventricles (spaces) within the brain.

Connected with the brain are 12 pairs of **cranial nerves**, most of which supply structures in the head. Most of these, like all the spinal nerves, are mixed nerves containing both sensory and motor fibers. A few of the cranial nerves contain only sensory fibers, whereas others are motor in function.

Addressing the Learning Outcomes

1. GIVE THE LOCATION OF THE FOUR MAIN DIVISIONS OF THE BRAIN.

EXERCISE 9-1: Brain, Sagittal Section (Text Fig. 9-1)

1. Write the names of the four labeled brain divisions in lines 1 to 4, using four different colors. Use red for #2 and blue for #3. DO NOT COLOR THE DIAGRAM YET.
2. Write the name of each labeled structure on the appropriate numbered line in different colors. Use different shades of red for structures 5 and 6 and different shades of blue for structures 8 to 10.
3. Color each structure on the diagram with the appropriate color.

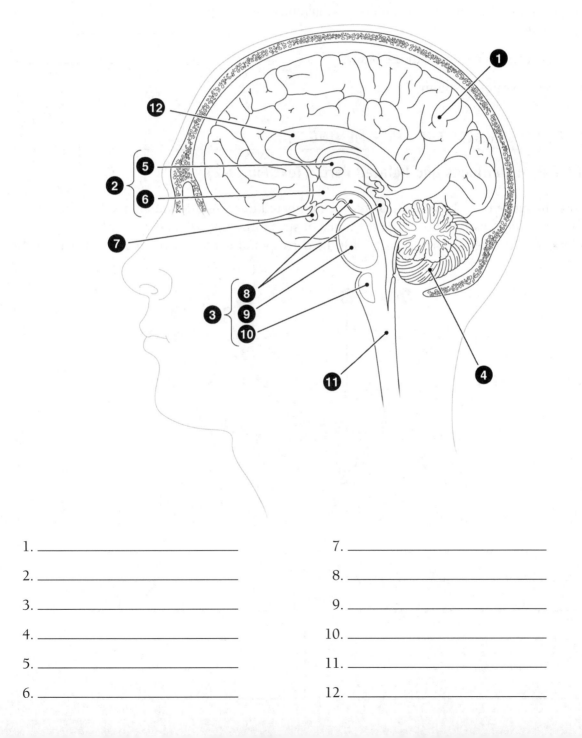

1. _____   7. _____

2. _____   8. _____

3. _____   9. _____

4. _____   10. _____

5. _____   11. _____

6. _____   12. _____

EXERCISE 9-2

Write the appropriate term in each blank from the list below.

lobe   hemisphere   cerebrum   diencephalon

brainstem   cerebellum

1. Each half of the cerebrum   _____

2. The "little" brain that coordinates voluntary muscle movements   _____

3. An individual subdivision of the cerebrum that regulates specific functions   _____

4. The portion of the brain that contains the thalamus and hypothalamus   _____

5. Connects the spinal cord with the brain   _____

6. The largest part of the brain   _____

2. NAME AND DESCRIBE THE THREE MENINGES.

EXERCISE 9-3: Meninges and Related Parts (Text Fig. 9-2)

1. Write the name of each labeled part on the numbered lines in different colors. Use the same color for structures 7 and 8. Write the name of structures 4, 9, 10, and 12 in black.
2. Color the structures on the diagram with the corresponding color. Do not color structures 4, 9, 10, and 12.

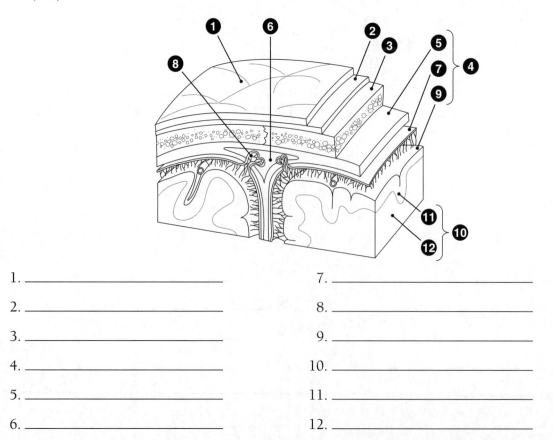

1. _____   7. _____

2. _____   8. _____

3. _____   9. _____

4. _____   10. _____

5. _____   11. _____

6. _____   12. _____

3. CITE THE FUNCTION OF CEREBROSPINAL FLUID AND DESCRIBE WHERE AND HOW THIS FLUID IS FORMED.

EXERCISE 9-4: Flow of Cerebrospinal Fluid (Text Fig. 9-3)

1. Write the name of each labeled part on the numbered lines in different colors. Use light colors for structures 5 to 12.
2. Color the structures on the diagram with the corresponding color. The boundaries between structures 5 to 12 (inclusive) are not always well defined. For instance, structure 6 is continuous with structure 7. You can overlap your colors to signify this fact.
3. Draw arrows to indicate the direction of CSF flow.

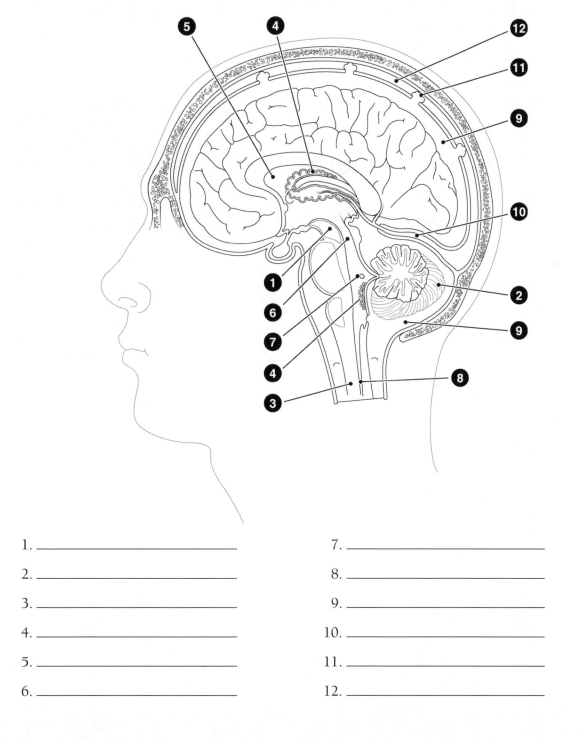

1. _____

2. _____

3. _____

4. _____

5. _____

6. _____

7. _____

8. _____

9. _____

10. _____

11. _____

12. _____

EXERCISE 9-5: Ventricles of the Brain (Text Fig. 9-4)

1. Write the name of each labeled part on the numbered lines in different colors. Write the names of structures 4, 5, and 6 in black because they will not be colored.

2. Color the structures on the diagram with the corresponding color (except for structures 4, 5, and 6). The boundaries between structures are not always well defined. For instance, structure 7 is continuous with structure 8. You can overlap your colors to signify this fact.

1. _____

2. _____

3. _____

4. _____

5. _____

6. _____

7. _____

8. _____

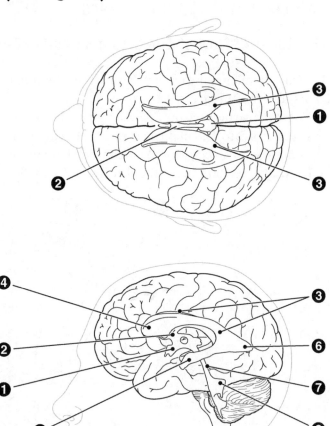

EXERCISE 9-6

Write the appropriate term in each blank from the list below.

dura mater   pia mater   arachnoid   choroid plexus

subarachnoid space   arachnoid villi   ventricle   dural sinus

cerebral aqueduct

1. The weblike middle meningeal layer   _____

2. Venous channel between the two outermost meninges   _____

3. The innermost layer of the meninges, the delicate membrane in which there are many blood vessels   _____

4. The area in which cerebrospinal fluid collects before its return to the blood   _____

5. The vascular network in a ventricle that forms cerebrospinal fluid   _____

6. The projections in the dural sinuses through which CSF is returned to the blood   _____

7. The outermost layer of the meninges, which is the thickest and the toughest   _____

4. NAME AND LOCATE THE LOBES OF THE CEREBRAL HEMISPHERES.

(Also see Exercise 9-8)

EXERCISE 9-7

Write the appropriate term in each blank from the list below.

gyrus   central sulcus   lateral sulcus   basal ganglia

dopamine   corpus callosum   internal capsule   cortex

1. A shallow groove that separates the temporal lobe from the frontal and parietal lobes   _____

2. Masses of gray matter deep within the cerebrum that help regulate body movement and the muscles of facial expression   _____

3. A band of white matter that carries impulses between the cerebrum and the brainstem   _____

4. An elevated portion of the cerebral cortex   _____

5. The thin layer of gray matter on the surface of the cerebrum   _____

6. A band of myelinated fibers that bridges the two cerebral hemispheres   _____

7. The neurotransmitter used by the basal nuclei neurons   _____

5. CITE ONE FUNCTION OF THE CEREBRAL CORTEX IN EACH LOBE OF THE CEREBRUM.

EXERCISE 9-8: Functional Areas of the Cerebral Cortex (Text Fig. 9-6)

1. Color the boxes next to the cerebral lobe names as follows: frontal lobe, pink; parietal lobe, light purple; temporal lobe, light blue; occipital lobe, light green.
2. Lightly color the four cerebral lobes on the diagram with the appropriate colors.
3. Write the names of structures 1 to 10 on the appropriate lines in different colors. For all structures except for #3, use a darker color than the one used for the corresponding cerebral lobe. For instance, a structure found in the frontal lobe could be colored red. Use the same color for structures 6 to 8. Use a dark color for structure 3.
4. Color or outline the structures on the diagram with the corresponding color.

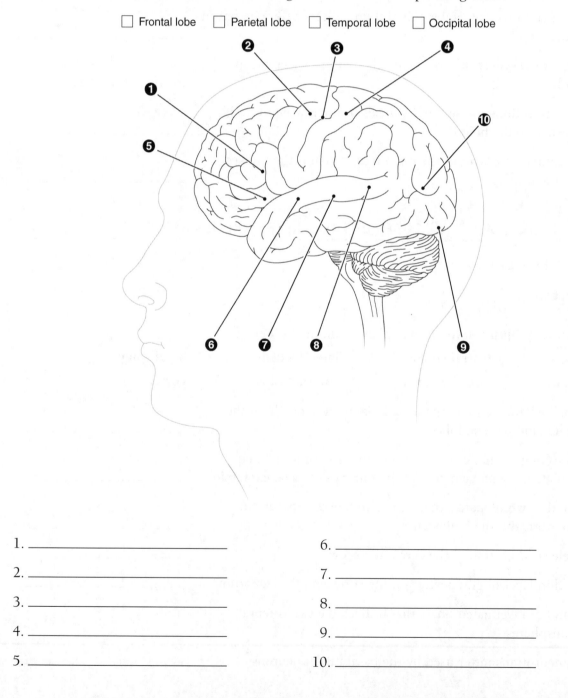

☐ Frontal lobe   ☐ Parietal lobe   ☐ Temporal lobe   ☐ Occipital lobe

1. _____   6. _____

2. _____   7. _____

3. _____   8. _____

4. _____   9. _____

5. _____   10. _____

EXERCISE 9-9

Write the appropriate term in each blank from the list below.

temporal lobe   parietal lobe   occipital lobe   frontal lobe

1. The portion of the cerebral cortex where visual impulses from the retina are interpreted

   _____

2. The portion of the cerebral cortex where auditory impulses are interpreted

   _____

3. Location of a sensory area for interpretation of pain, touch, and temperature

   _____

4. The lobe controlling voluntary muscles

   _____

6. NAME TWO DIVISIONS OF THE DIENCEPHALON AND CITE THE FUNCTIONS OF EACH.

See Exercise 9-10.

7. LOCATE THE THREE SUBDIVISIONS OF THE BRAINSTEM AND GIVE THE FUNCTIONS OF EACH.

EXERCISE 9-10

Write the appropriate term in each blank from the list below.

thalamus   pons   midbrain   hypothalamus

vasomotor center   medulla oblongata   cardiac center   limbic system

1. The portion of the brainstem composed of myelinated nerve fibers that connects to the cerebellum

   _____

2. The superior portion of the brainstem

   _____

3. The part of the brain between the pons and the spinal cord

   _____

4. The region of the diencephalon that acts as a relay center for sensory stimuli

   _____

5. The region consisting of portions of the cerebrum and diencephalon that is involved in emotional states and behavior

   _____

6. Nuclei that regulate the contraction of smooth muscle in blood vessel walls

   _____

7. The portion of the brain controlling the autonomic nervous system

   _____

8. DESCRIBE THE CEREBELLUM AND IDENTIFY ITS FUNCTIONS.

EXERCISE 9-11

List three functions of the cerebellum in the spaces below.

1. _____

2. _____

3. _____

9. DESCRIBE FOUR TECHNIQUES USED TO STUDY THE BRAIN.

EXERCISE 9-12

Write the appropriate term in each blank from the list below.

MRI   CT   PET   EEG

1. Technique that produces a picture of brain activity levels in
   the different parts of the brain   _____

2. Technique that measures electric currents in the brain   _____

3. X-ray technique that provides photos of bone, cavities,
   and lesions   _____

4. Technique used to visualize soft tissue, such as scar tissue,
   hemorrhages, and tumors that does not use X-rays   _____

10. LIST THE NAMES AND FUNCTIONS OF THE 12 CRANIAL NERVES.

EXERCISE 9-13: Cranial Nerves (Text Fig. 9-11)

1. Write the number and name of each labeled cranial nerve on the numbered lines in different colors. Use the same color for structures 1 and 2.
2. Color the nerves on the diagram with the corresponding color.

1. _____
2. _____
3. _____
4. _____
5. _____
6. _____
7. _____
8. _____
9. _____
10. _____
11. _____
12. _____
13. _____

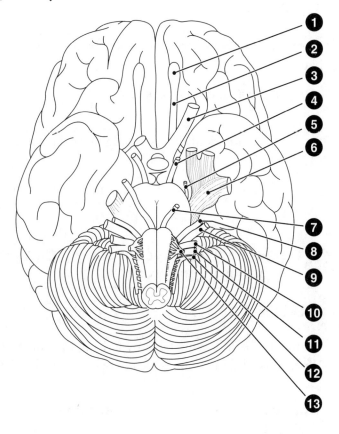

EXERCISE 9-14

Write the appropriate term in each blank from the list below.

optic nerve	glossopharyngeal nerve	trochlear nerve
abducens nerve	vagus nerve	vestibulocochlear nerve
facial nerve	trigeminal nerve	accessory nerve

1. A motor nerve controlling the trapezius, sternocleidomastoid, and larynx muscles _____

2. The nerve that controls contraction of a single eye muscle _____

3. The nerve that carries visual impulses from the eye to the brain _____

4. The most important sensory nerve of the face and the head _____

5. The nerve that supplies most of the organs in the thoracic and the abdominal cavities _____

6. The nerve that supplies the muscles of facial expression _____

7. The nerve that carries sensory impulses for hearing and equilibrium _____

11. MATCH SOME OF THE PATIENT'S SIGNS AND SYMPTOMS IN THE CASE STUDY TO THE PARTS OF HIS BRAIN THAT WERE DAMAGED BY THE STROKE.

EXERCISE 9-15

Match the following problems with the damaged brain area by writing the appropriate letter in the blank.

_____ 1. slurred, difficult speech

_____ 2. weakness of the right side of his face and arm

_____ 3. loss of sensation from the right side of his face and arm

a. primary motor area, frontal lobe

b. motor speech area, frontal lobe, left hemisphere

c. primary sensory area, parietal lobe

12. SHOW HOW WORD PARTS ARE USED TO BUILD WORDS RELATED TO THE NERVOUS SYSTEM.

EXERCISE 9-16

Complete the following table by writing the correct word part or meaning in the space provided. Write a word that contains each word part in the "Example" column.

Word Part	Meaning	Example
1. _____	cut	_____
2. chori/o	_____	_____
3. _____	tongue	_____
4. encephal/o	_____	_____
5. cerebr/o	_____	_____
6. _____	opposed, against	_____
7. _____	lateral, side	_____
8. gyr/o	_____	_____

Making the Connections

The following concept map deals with brain anatomy. Complete the concept map by filling in the appropriate term or phrase that describes the indicated structure.

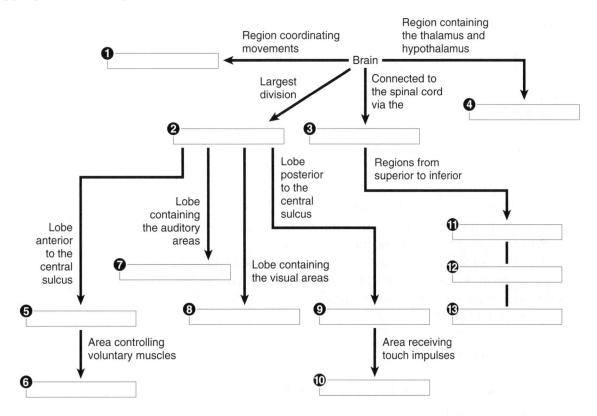

Optional Exercise: Make your own concept map based on structures involved in the synthesis and movement of CSF. Choose your own terms to incorporate into your map, or use the following list: ventricle, choroid plexus, lateral ventricles, third ventricle, fourth ventricle, foramina, horns, cerebral aqueduct, spinal cord, hydrocephalus, CSF, dural sinuses, subarachnoid space, arachnoid villi.

Testing Your Knowledge

BUILDING UNDERSTANDING

I. MULTIPLE CHOICE

Select the best answer and write the letter of your choice in the blank.

1. What is the name of the shallow groove separating the frontal and parietal lobes?
   a. lateral sulcus
   b. central sulcus
   c. longitudinal fissure
   d. basal nuclei

   1. _____

2. Which of these phrases describes the dura mater?
   a. the innermost layer of the meninges
   b. the outermost layer of the meninges
   c. the network of vessels that produces cerebrospinal fluid
   d. the part of the brain that connects with the spinal cord

   2. _____

3. Which brain region receives visual impulses?
   a. parietal lobe
   b. temporal lobe
   c. hippocampus
   d. occipital lobe

   3. _____

4. Which of these structures *forms* cerebrospinal fluid?
   a. cerebral aqueduct
   b. central sulcus
   c. choroid plexus
   d. internal capsule

   4. _____

5. Which of these regions is innervated by the abducens nerve?
   a. eye
   b. ear and pharynx
   c. face and salivary gland
   d. tongue and pharynx

   5. _____

6. Which groove separates the frontal and parietal lobes of each hemisphere?
   a. lateral sulcus
   b. central sulcus
   c. medial sulcus
   d. superior sulcus

   6. _____

7. What is the reticular formation?
   a. a region of the limbic system that controls wakefulness and sleep
   b. a deep groove that divides the cerebral hemispheres
   c. the part of the temporal lobe concerned with the sense of smell
   d. the fifth lobe of the cerebrum

   7. _____

II. COMPLETION EXERCISE

Write the word or the phrase that correctly completes each sentence.

1. The ventricle posterior to the brainstem and anterior to the cerebellum is the

   _____.

2. The four chambers within the brain where cerebrospinal fluid is produced are the

   _____.

3. Sounds are interpreted in the area of the temporal lobe called the _____.

4. The region of the diencephalon that helps maintain homeostasis (e.g., water balance, appetite, and body temperature) and controls the autonomic nervous system is the

   _____.

5. The hypothalamic nucleus controlling the muscle in blood vessel walls is called the

   _____.

6. Records of the electrical activity of the brain can be made with an instrument called a(n)

   _____.

7. Extensions of the lateral ventricles into the cerebral lobes are called

   _____.

8. Except for the first two pairs, all the cranial nerves arise from the _____.

9. The three layers of membranes that surround the brain and spinal cord are called the

   _____.

10. The clear liquid that helps to support and protect the brain and spinal cord is

    _____.

11. The number of pairs of cranial nerves is _____.

12. The widespread collection of brain tissue involved in emotion and memories is called the

    _____.

13. The middle portion of the cerebellum is called the _____.

UNDERSTANDING CONCEPTS

I. TRUE/FALSE

For each question, write T for true or F for false in the blank to the left of each number. If a statement is false, correct it by replacing the underlined term and write the correct statement in the blanks below the question.

_____ 1. The pia mater is the middle layer of the meninges.

_____

_____ 2. The interventricular foramina form channels between the lateral ventricles and the fourth ventricle.

_____

_____ 3. The primary motor cortex is found in the parietal lobe.

_____

_____ 4. The internal capsule consists of myelinated fibers linking the cerebral hemispheres with the brainstem.

_____

_____ 5. The reticular activating system governs alertness and sleep.

_____

_____ 6. The raised areas on the surface of the cerebrum are called gyri.

_____

_____ 7. Auditory (sound) impulses are carried by the third cranial nerve.

_____

_____ 8. The hypoglossal nerve transmits sensory information from the tongue.

_____

II. PRACTICAL APPLICATIONS

Study each discussion. Then write the appropriate word or phrase in the space provided.

1. Mr. B, aged 87, drove his car into a ditch. When the paramedics arrived, he was unable to speak. The paramedics suspected damage to the cerebral lobe containing the motor speech area. This lobe is the _____.

2. Mr. B also experienced paralysis on his right side, indicating a problem within the largest division of the brain, the _____.

3. The damaged brain region controlling voluntary movements is called the _____.

4. The right side of Mr. B's face droops, and he cannot control his facial expressions. The facial muscles are controlled by the cranial nerve numbered _____.

5. A ruptured blood vessel was observed using a CT scan. CT is an abbreviation for
_____.

6. The rupture occurred in the left side of the brain. The anatomical name for the left side of the brain is the left _____.

7. Mr. B's speech disorder indicates that the bleed affected his motor speech area, also called
_____.

III. SHORT ESSAYS

1. Describe the structures that protect the brain and spinal cord.

_____

_____

_____

2. List some functions of the structures in the diencephalon.

_____

_____

_____

3. List the name, number, and sensory information conveyed for each of the purely sensory cranial nerves.

_____

_____

_____

_____

_____

CONCEPTUAL THINKING

1. Describe the journey of CSF, beginning with its synthesis and ending with its entry into the circulatory system.

_____

_____

_____

_____

_____

Expanding Your Horizons

Do you use herbal supplements like ginko biloba to boost your learning power? As discussed in this *Scientific American* article (Gold PE, Cahill L, Wenk GL. The lowdown on Ginkgo biloba. Sci Am 2003;288:86–91), ginko biloba does boost memory—to the same extent as a candy bar! Mental exercise may be the best way to improve your academic performance (Holloway M. The mutable brain. Sci Am 2003;289:78–85).

CHAPTER

10

The Sensory System

Overview

The sensory system enables us to detect changes taking place both internally and externally. These changes are detected by specialized structures called **sensory receptors**. Any change that acts on a receptor to induce a nerve impulse is termed a stimulus. The special senses, so called because the receptors are limited to a few specialized sense organs in the head, include the senses of vision, hearing, equilibrium, taste, and smell. The receptors of the eye are the rods and cones located in the retina. The receptors for both hearing (the spiral organ) and equilibrium (the vestibule and semicircular canals) are located within the inner ear. Receptors for the chemical senses of taste and smell are located on the tongue and in the upper part of the nose, respectively. The general senses are scattered throughout the body; they respond to touch, pressure, temperature, pain, and position. Receptors for the sense of position, known as proprioceptors, are found in muscles, tendons, and joints. The nerve impulses generated by a receptor in response to a stimulus must be carried to the central nervous system by way of a sensory (afferent) neuron. Here, the information is processed and a suitable response is made.

   This chapter is quite challenging, because it contains both difficult concepts and large amounts of detail. You can use concept maps to assemble all of the details into easy-to-remember frameworks.

Addressing the Learning Outcomes

1. DESCRIBE THE FUNCTION OF THE SENSORY SYSTEM.

EXERCISE 10-1

Fill in the blanks in the following paragraph using these terms:
central nervous system, homeostasis, sensory neuron, sensory receptor

The sensory system protects people by detecting changes in the internal and external environments that threaten to disrupt (1) _____, which is the maintenance of a constant internal environment. The change is detected by a (2) _____, which sends an impulse through a (3) _____ to the (4) _____.

2. DIFFERENTIATE BETWEEN THE DIFFERENT TYPES OF SENSORY RECEPTORS AND GIVE EXAMPLES OF EACH.

EXERCISE 10-2

Classify each of the following senses as general senses (G) or special senses (S).

1. Sense of position _____

2. Smell _____

3. Vision _____

4. Touch _____

5. Temperature _____

6. Equilibrium _____

3. DESCRIBE SENSORY ADAPTATION AND EXPLAIN ITS VALUE.

EXERCISE 10-3

Define *sensory adaptation* in the space below.

_____

_____

4. LIST AND DESCRIBE THE STRUCTURES THAT PROTECT THE EYE.

EXERCISE 10-4: The Lacrimal Apparatus (Text Fig. 10-2)

Label the indicated parts.

1. _____

2. _____

3. _____

4. _____

5. _____

6. _____

7. _____

5. IDENTIFY THE THREE TUNICS OF THE EYE.

EXERCISE 10-5: The Eye (Text Fig. 10-3)

1. Color the small boxes yellow (nervous tunic), red, (vascular tunic) and blue (fibrous tunic).
2. Write the name of each labeled part on the numbered lines in different colors. Follow this color scheme:
   - Yellow: 6, 7, 8, and 9
   - Red: 5, 10, 11, 13
   - Blue: 3, 4
   - Choose your own colors for the other structures.
3. Color the different structures on the diagram with the corresponding color. Some structures are present in more than one location on the diagram. Try to color all of a particular structure in the appropriate color. For instance, only one of the suspensory ligaments is labeled, but color both suspensory ligaments.

☐ Nervous tunic   ☐ Vascular tunic   ☐ Fibrous tunic

1. _____
2. _____
3. _____
4. _____
5. _____
6. _____
7. _____
8. _____

9. _____
10. _____
11. _____
12. _____
13. _____
14. _____
15. _____
16. _____

6. DEFINE *REFRACTION* AND LIST THE REFRACTIVE PARTS OF THE EYE.

EXERCISE 10-6

List four eye structures that bend (refract) light in the spaces below.

1. _____
2. _____
3. _____
4. _____

7. DIFFERENTIATE BETWEEN THE RODS AND THE CONES OF THE EYE.

EXERCISE 10-7

Write the appropriate term in each blank from the list below.

cone   cornea   rhodopsin   sclera

optic disk   retina   rod   fovea centralis

1. A vision receptor that is sensitive to color _____

2. The part of the eye that light rays pass through first as they enter the eye _____

3. Another name for the blind spot, the region where the optic nerve connects with the eye _____

4. The innermost coat of the eyeball, the nervous tissue layer that includes the receptors for the sense of vision _____

5. A vision receptor that functions well in dim light _____

6. A pigment needed for vision _____

7. The depressed area in the retina that is the point of clearest vision _____

8. COMPARE THE FUNCTIONS OF THE EXTRINSIC AND THE INTRINSIC EYE MUSCLES.

EXERCISE 10-8: Extrinsic Muscles of the Eye (Text Fig. 10-6)

1. Write the name of each labeled muscle on the numbered lines in different colors.
2. Color the different muscles on the diagram with the corresponding color.

1. _____

2. _____

3. _____

4. _____

5. _____

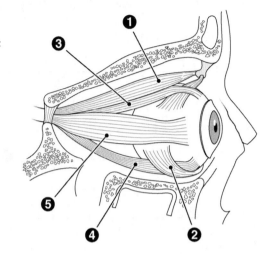

EXERCISE 10-9

Write the appropriate term in each blank from the list below.

aqueous humor **vitreous body** **lens** **ciliary muscle**

choroid **conjunctiva** **pupil** **iris**

1. The structure that alters the shape of the lens for accommodation

   _____

2. The watery fluid that fills much of the eyeball in front of the crystalline lens

   _____

3. The vascular, pigmented middle tunic of the eyeball

   _____

4. Structure with two sets of muscle fibers that regulate the amount of light entering the eye

   _____

5. The jellylike material located behind the crystalline lens that maintains the spherical shape of the eyeball

   _____

6. The central opening of the iris

   _____

7. The membrane that lines the eyelids

   _____

9. DESCRIBE THE NERVE SUPPLY TO THE EYE.

Also see Exercise 10-17.

EXERCISE 10-10: Nerves of the Eye (Text Fig. 10-10)

Label the indicated nerves.

1. _____

2. _____

3. _____

4. _____

5. _____

6. _____

10. DESCRIBE THE THREE DIVISIONS OF THE EAR.

EXERCISE 10-11: The Ear (Text Fig. 10-11)

1. Write the names of the three ear divisions on the appropriate lines (1 to 3).
2. Write the names of the labeled parts on the numbered lines in different colors. Use black for structures 12 to 14 because they will not be colored.
3. Color each part with the corresponding color (except for parts 12 to 14).

1. _____

2. _____

3. _____

4. _____

5. _____

6. _____

7. _____

8. _____

9. _____

10. _____

11. _____

12. _____

13. _____

14. _____

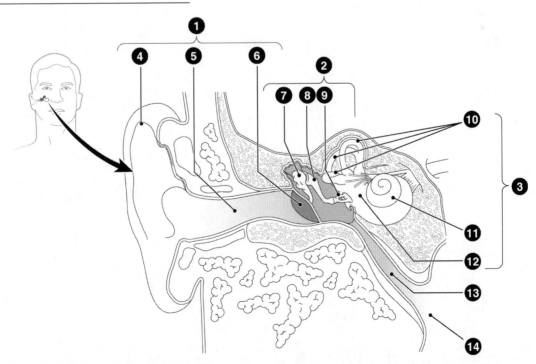

EXERCISE 10-12: The Inner Ear (Text Fig. 10-12)

Label the indicated parts.

1. _____

2. _____

3. _____

4. _____

5. _____

6. _____

7. _____

8. _____

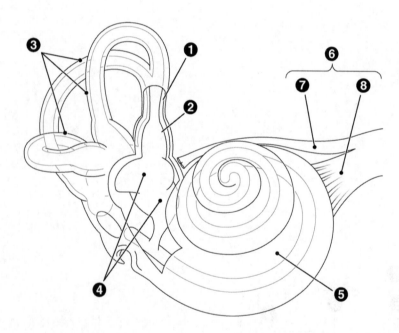

11. DESCRIBE THE RECEPTOR FOR HEARING AND EXPLAIN HOW IT FUNCTIONS.

EXERCISE 10-13: Cochlea and Spiral Organ (Text Fig. 10-13)

1. Write the name of each labeled part on the numbered lines. Use colors for structures 3 to 7, 11, and 12. Use black for the other structures. Bullets 8 and 9 indicate fluids.
2. Color structures 3 to 7, 11, and 12 with the corresponding color. Try to color all of a particular structure in the appropriate color. For example, the cochlear duct is labeled once but is visible in three places.

1. _____
2. _____
3. _____
4. _____
5. _____
6. _____
7. _____
8. _____
9. _____
10. _____
11. _____
12. _____
13. _____

EXERCISE 10-14

Write the appropriate term in each blank from the list below.

oval window   spiral organ   malleus
eustachian tube   cochlear duct   endolymph
perilymph   incus   pinna

1. The fluid contained within the membranous labyrinth of the inner ear   _____

2. The bone in contact with the tympanic membrane   _____

3. Another name for the projecting part, or auricle, of the ear   _____

4. The channel connecting the middle ear cavity with the pharynx _____

5. The fluid of the inner ear contained within the bony labyrinth and surrounding the membranous labyrinth   _____

6. The structure containing the receptor cells for hearing   _____

7. The skeleton of the inner ear   _____

8. The duct in the spiral organ that contains endolymph   _____

12. COMPARE THE LOCATION AND FUNCTION OF THE EQUILIBRIUM RECEPTORS.

EXERCISE 10-15

Write the appropriate term in each blank from the list below.

vestibule   macula   crista   semicircular canal
cochlear duct   hair cells   otoliths

1. Ciliated cells found in both the vestibule and the semicircular canals   _____

2. Small crystals that help activate maculae   _____

3. One of three chambers that detect rotation   _____

4. A structure containing hair cells and a cupula   _____

5. Two small chambers containing maculae   _____

6. The collection of hair cells found in a vestibule   _____

13. DISCUSS THE LOCATION AND FUNCTION OF THE SPECIAL SENSE ORGANS FOR TASTE AND SMELL.

EXERCISE 10-16

Replace the underlined terms in each of the following statements to make each statement true.

a. The sense of smell is <u>gustation</u> and the sense of taste is <u>olfaction</u>.

_____

b. Substances to be smelled and tasted must always be <u>free in the air</u> surrounding the receptor cell.

_____

c. We have hundreds of different types of <u>taste receptors</u> but less than ten types of <u>odor receptors</u>.

_____

d. Organic compounds activate <u>sour receptors</u> and hydrogen ions activate <u>salty receptors</u>.

_____

14. EXPLAIN THE FUNCTION OF PROPRIOCEPTORS.

EXERCISE 10-17

Write the appropriate term in each blank from the list below.

kinesthesia   proprioception   tactile corpuscle   cochlear nerve

vestibular nerve   oculomotor nerve   ophthalmic nerve

optic nerve   free nerve endings   equilibrium

1. The branch of the vestibulocochlear nerve that carries hearing impulses

_____

2. The nerve that carries visual impulses from the retina to the brain

_____

3. The branch of the fifth cranial nerve that carries impulses of pain, touch, and temperature from the eye to the brain

_____

4. The largest of the three cranial nerves that carry motor fibers to the eyeball muscles

_____

5. The sense of knowing the position of one's body and the relative positions of different muscles

_____

6. The sense of body movement

_____

7. Receptors that detect changes in temperature

_____

8. The semicircular canals are involved in this sense

_____

15. USING THE CASE, DISCUSS CHANGES IN THE ANATOMY AND PHYSIOLOGY OF THE EYE RESULTING FROM CHRONIC SUN EXPOSURE.

EXERCISE 10-18

In the lines below, explain how sunlight affects (a) the lens and (b) the retina.

a. _____

_____

b. _____

_____

16. SHOW HOW WORD PARTS ARE USED TO BUILD WORDS RELATED TO THE SENSORY SYSTEM.

EXERCISE 10-19

Complete the following table by writing the correct word part or meaning in the space provided. Write a word that contains each word part in the Example column.

Word Part	Meaning	Example
1. kine	_____	_____
2. _____	stone	_____
3. ot/o	_____	_____
4. ophthalm/o	_____	_____
5. _____	drum	_____
6. _____	yellow	_____
7. propri/o	_____	_____
8. -esthesia	_____	_____

Making the Connections

The following concept map deals with the structure and function of the eye. Each pair of terms is linked together by a connecting phrase into a sentence. The sentence should be read in the direction of the arrow. Complete the concept map by filling in the appropriate term or phrase. There is one right answer for each term. However, there are many correct answers for the connecting phrases (2, 9).

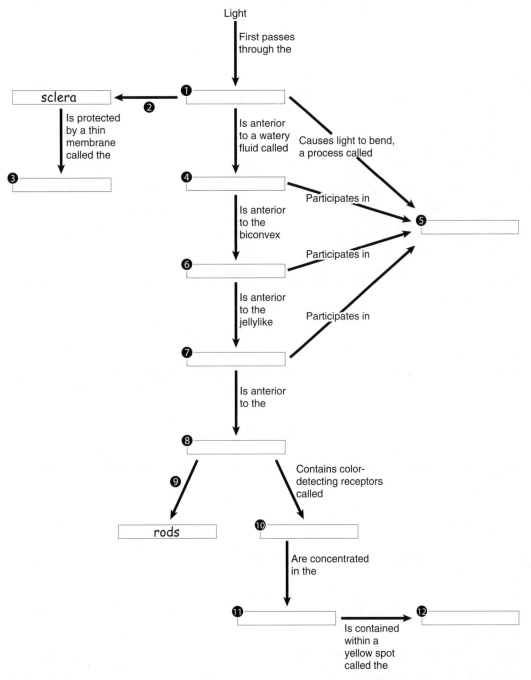

Optional Exercise: Construct a concept map of terms relating to the ear using the following terms and any others you would like to include: tympanic membrane, stapes, malleus, incus, pinna, bony labyrinth, spiral organ, oval window, round window, cochlear duct, tectorial membrane, cochlear nerve. You may also want to construct concept maps relating to the other special senses (equilibrium, taste, smell) and the general senses (touch, pressure, temperature, proprioception).

Testing Your Knowledge

BUILDING UNDERSTANDING

I. MULTIPLE CHOICE

1. Which of the following receptor types responds to light?
   a. photoreceptor
   b. mechanoreceptor
   c. chemoreceptor
   d. thermoreceptor

1. _____

2. Which of the following terms relates to the sense of touch?
   a. tactile
   b. gustatory
   c. proprioceptive
   d. thermal

2. _____

3. What process alters the lens' shape to allow for near or far vision?
   a. accommodation
   b. convergence
   c. divergence
   d. dark adaptation

3. _____

4. Which secretion is involved in the process of *lacrimation*?
   a. mucus
   b. wax
   c. tears
   d. aqueous humor

4. _____

5. Which of these bones is in contact with the tympanic membrane?
   a. incus
   b. malleus
   c. stapes
   d. pinna

5. _____

6. Which of these structures is the transparent part of the fibrous tunic?
   a. sclera
   b. cornea
   c. conjunctiva
   d. choroid

6. _____

7. Which of the following is the receptor for hearing?
   a. spiral organ
   b. macula
   c. olfactory bulb
   d. retina

7. _____

8. Which of these structures detects temperature?
   a. proprioceptor
   b. olfactory receptor
   c. mechanoreceptor
   d. free nerve ending

8. _____

9. Which of the following is a component of the eye's vascular tunic?   9. _____
    a. retina
    b. cornea
    c. choroid
    d. lens
10. Which of the following structures is involved in sensing gravity?   10. _____
    a. cupula
    b. vestibular duct
    c. otoliths
    d. crista

II. COMPLETION EXERCISE

1. The transparent portion of the sclera is the _____.

2. The glands that secrete earwax are called _____.

3. The receptors that aid in judging position and changes in location of body parts are the _____.

4. The sense of position is partially governed by equilibrium receptors in the internal ear, including two small chambers in the vestibule and the three _____.

5. The ciliated cells that function in hearing and equilibrium are called

   _____.

6. All sensory receptors that respond to light all called _____.

7. When you enter a darkened room, it takes a while for the rods to begin to function. This interval is known as the period of _____.

8. The nervous tunic of the eye is the _____.

9. The muscles that adjust the shape of the lens are called _____.

UNDERSTANDING CONCEPTS

I. TRUE/FALSE

For each question, write T for true or F for false in the blank to the left of each number. If a statement is false, correct it by replacing the underlined term and write the correct statement in the blanks below the question.

_____ 1. Extrinsic eye muscles control the diameter of the pupil.

_____

_____ 2. A crista contains receptor (hair) cells and a gelatinous otolith membrane.

_____

_____ 3. The incus is in contact with the oval window of the inner ear.

_____

_____ 4. The cochlear duct contains <u>endolymph</u>.

_____

_____ 5. The <u>rods</u> of the eye function in bright light and detect color.

_____

_____ 6. When the eyes are exposed to a bright light, the pupils <u>constrict.</u>

_____

_____ 7. The <u>ophthalmic</u> nerve carries visual impulses from the retina to the brain.

_____

_____ 8. The ciliary muscle <u>contracts</u> to thicken the lens.

_____

_____ 9. The sense of smell is also called <u>olfaction.</u>

_____

II. PRACTICAL APPLICATIONS

Study each discussion. Then write the appropriate word or phrase in the space provided.

➤ Group A

Baby L was brought in by his mother because he awakened crying and holding the right side of his head. He had been suffering from a cold, but now he seemed to be in pain. Complete the following descriptions relating to his evaluation and treatment.

1. Examination revealed a bulging red eardrum. The eardrum is also called the
   _____.

2. The cause of baby L's painful bulging eardrum was an infection of the middle ear. The middle ear contains three small bones, collectively known as the _____.

3. Antibiotic treatment of baby L's middle ear infection was begun, because this early treatment usually prevents complications. The middle ear is prone to infections, because it is connected to the pharynx by the _____.

4. Baby L was returned to the emergency room the next day because he was falling down repeatedly. The physician suspected a problem with his sense of balance, or
   _____.

5. Baby L's mother asked how an ear infection could affect balance. The physician explained that two structures were located within the inner ear that are involved with balance, named the semicircular canals and the _____.

6. In particular, the physician feared that the middle ear infection had spread to the fluid within the membranous labyrinth. This fluid is called _____.

➤ **Group B**

Sixty-year old Mr. S had ridden his scooter over some broken glass. A fragment of glass bounced up and flew into one eye. Complete the following descriptions relating to his evaluation and treatment.

1. Examination by the eye specialist showed that there was a cut in the transparent window of the eye, the _____.

2. On further examination of Mr. S, the colored part of the eye was seen to protrude from the wound. This part of the eye is the _____.

3. Mr. S's treatment included antiseptics, anesthetics, and suturing of the wound. Medication was instilled in the saclike structure at the anterior of the eyeball. This sac is lined with a thin epithelial membrane, the _____.

➤ **Group C**

You are conducting hearing tests at a senior citizens' home. During the course of the afternoon, you encounter the following patients. Complete the following descriptions relating to the ear structure and function.

1. Mrs. B complained of some hearing loss and a sense of fullness in her outer ear. Examination revealed that her ear canal was plugged with hardened ear wax, which is scientifically called _____.

2. Mr. J, age 72, complained of gradually worsening hearing loss, although he had no symptoms of pain or other ear problems. Examination revealed that his hearing loss was due to nerve damage. The cranial nerve that carries hearing impulses to the brain is called the _____.

3. In particular, the endings of this nerve were damaged. These nerve endings are located in the spiral-shaped part of the inner ear, a part of the ear that is known as the _____.

III. SHORT ESSAYS

1. Describe several different structural forms of sensory receptors and give examples of each.

_____

_____

_____

2. Hair cells function as receptor cells in three different sensory organs. Compare and contrast these three sensory organs by completing the following table. Some boxes have been filled in for you.

Sensory Organ Name	Membrane Overlying Hair Cell	Stimulus Sensed by the Sensory Organ
		Gravity and linear acceleration
	Tectorial membrane	
Crista		

CONCEPTUAL THINKING

1. You have probably been sitting in a chair for quite a while, yet you have not been constantly aware of your legs contacting the chair. Why not?

_____

_____

_____

2. Write your name at the bottom of this sheet of paper. Explain the contributions of different sensory receptors that were required to successfully complete that simple task. For instance, proprioceptors are required to indicate where the fingers are each moment of time.

_____

_____

_____

Expanding Your Horizons

1. Imagine if you could taste a triangle, or hear blue. This is reality for individuals with a disorder called *synesthesia*. Read about some exceptional artists that suffer from this disorder, and how synthesia has helped us understand how the brain processes sensory information, in the article below. You can get a taste of how synesthetics view the world in the exercises at the Web site listed below.

   • Ramachandran VS, Hubbard EM. Hearing colors, tasting shapes. Sci Am 2003;288:52–59.
   • Synesthesia and the Synesthetic Experience. Available at: http://web.mit.edu/synesthesia/www/

2. Here is an exercise you can do to find your own blind spot. Draw a cross (on the left) and a circle (on the right) on a piece of paper that are separated by a hand width. Focus on the cross, and notice (but do not focus on) the circle. Move the paper closer and further away until the circle disappears. Weird activities to investigate your blind spot can be found at this Web site:

   • The Blind Spot Test. Available at: http://www.blindspottest.com/

CHAPTER

11

The Endocrine System: Glands and Hormones

Overview

The endocrine system and the nervous system are the main coordinating and controlling systems of the body. Chapters 8 and 9 discuss how the nervous system uses chemical and electrical stimuli to control very rapid, short-term responses. This chapter discusses the endocrine system, which uses specific chemicals called hormones to induce short-term or long-term changes in the reproduction, development, and function of specific cells. Although some hormones act locally, most travel in the blood to distant sites and exert their effects on any cell (the target cell) that contains a specific receptor for the hormone. Although hormones are produced by many tissues, certain glands, called endocrine glands, specialize in hormone production. These endocrine glands include the pituitary (hypophysis), thyroid, parathyroids, adrenals, pancreas, gonads, and pineal. Together, these glands comprise the endocrine system. The activity of endocrine glands is regulated by negative feedback, other hormones, nervous stimulation, and/or biological rhythms. One of the most important endocrine glands is the pituitary gland, which comprises the anterior pituitary and the posterior pituitary. The posterior pituitary gland is made of nervous tissue—it contains the axons and terminals of neurons that have their cell bodies in a part of the brain called the hypothalamus. Hormones are synthesized in the hypothalamus and released from the posterior pituitary. The anterior pituitary secretes a number of hormones that act on other endocrine glands. The cells of the anterior pituitary are controlled in part by releasing hormones made in the hypothalamus. These releasing hormones pass through the blood vessels of a portal circulation to reach the anterior pituitary. Hormones are also made outside the traditional endocrine glands. Other structures that secrete hormones include the stomach, small intestine, kidney, heart, skin, and placenta. Hormones are extremely potent, and small variations in hormone concentrations can have significant effects on the body.

This chapter contains a lot of details for you to learn. Try to summarize the material using concept maps and summary tables. You should also understand negative feedback (Chapter 1) before you tackle the concepts in this chapter.

Addressing the Learning Outcomes

1. COMPARE THE EFFECTS OF THE NERVOUS SYSTEM AND THE ENDOCRINE SYSTEM IN CONTROLLING THE BODY.

EXERCISE 11-1

Fill in the blank after each characteristic—to the nervous system (N) or the endocrine system (E)?

1. Controls rapid responses _____

2. Used to regulate growth _____

3. Uses chemical stimuli only _____

4. Uses both chemical and electrical stimuli _____

2. DESCRIBE THE FUNCTIONS OF HORMONES.

EXERCISE 11-2

Define the following terms:

1. Receptor _____

2. Target tissue _____

3. Hormone _____

3. DISCUSS THE CHEMICAL COMPOSITION OF HORMONES.

EXERCISE 11-3

Fill in the blank after each statement—does it apply to amino acid compounds (A) or lipids (L)?

1. Protein hormones _____

2. Can be formed by modifying cholesterol _____

3. Hormones of the sex glands and the adrenal cortex _____

4. Hormones not produced by the sex glands or the adrenal cortex _____

5. Prostaglandins _____

4. EXPLAIN HOW HORMONES ARE REGULATED.

EXERCISE 11-4

a. Define *negative feedback*.

_____

_____

b. Which of the situations below are examples of negative feedback? Circle all that apply.

   i. When the concentration of thyroid hormone in blood increases, the secretion of thyroid-stimulating hormone from the pituitary gland decreases.

   ii. When the concentration of growth hormone in blood increases, the production of growth hormone from the pituitary gland decreases.

   iii. When the house heats up, the furnace produces less heat.

   iv. When an astute investor makes money on a stock deal, he can make further investments to make even more money.

5. IDENTIFY THE GLANDS OF THE ENDOCRINE SYSTEM ON A DIAGRAM.

EXERCISE 11-5: The Endocrine Glands (Text Fig. 11-2)

1. Write the name of each labeled part on the numbered lines in different colors.
2. Color the different structures on the diagram with the corresponding color. Make sure you color all four parathyroid glands.

1. _____

2. _____

3. _____

4. _____

5. _____

6. _____

7. _____

8. _____

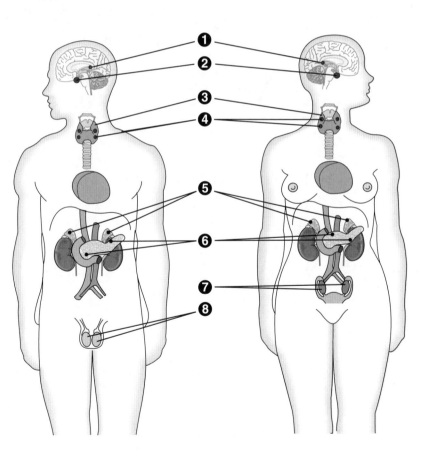

EXERCISE 11-6

Write the term in the appropriate blank from the list below.

parathyroid   pineal   hypothalamus

thyroid   adrenal   pancreas

1. One of the tiny glands located behind the thyroid gland   _____

2. The largest of the endocrine glands, located in the neck   _____

3. The gland in the brain that is regulated by light   _____

4. An organ that contains islets   _____

5. The endocrine gland composed of a cortex and medulla, each with specific functions   _____

6. LIST THE HORMONES PRODUCED BY EACH ENDOCRINE GLAND AND DESCRIBE THE EFFECTS OF EACH ON THE BODY.

EXERCISE 11-7

Fill in the missing information in the chart below. This table does not cover all of the hormones and their actions discussed in the text. Do not fill in the column at the far right yet. This column will be discussed under Outcome 9.

Hormone	Gland	Effects	Medical Uses
ADH (antidiuretic hormone)			N/A
	Adrenal cortex	Increases blood glucose concentration in response to stress	
		uterine contraction, milk ejection	
	Anterior pituitary	Promotes growth of all body tissues	
Parathyroid hormone			N/A
	Pancreas	Reduces blood glucose concentrations by promoting glucose uptake into cells and glucose storage; promotes fat and protein synthesis	
Thyroid hormones: thyroxine (T_4) and triiodothyronine (T_3)			
	Adrenal cortex	Promotes salt (and thus water) retention and potassium excretion	N/A
		Stimulates glucose release from the liver, thereby increasing blood glucose levels	N/A
Melatonin			N/A

EXERCISE 11-8

Write the appropriate term in each blank from the list below.

epinephrine   antidiuretic hormone   ACTH

follicle-stimulating hormone   estrogen

aldosterone   prolactin

1. The anterior pituitary hormone that stimulates milk synthesis   _____

2. The main hormone of the adrenal medulla that, among other actions, raises blood pressure and increases the heart rate   _____

3. The anterior pituitary hormone that stimulates the adrenal cortex   _____

4. A hormone produced by the ovaries   _____

5. The hormone from the adrenal cortex that regulates sodium and potassium reabsorption in the kidney tubules   _____

6. A gonadotropic hormone   _____

7. A hormone synthesized in the hypothalamus   _____

EXERCISE 11-9

Write the appropriate term in each blank from the list below.

insulin   glucagon   parathyroid hormone   testosterone   cortisol

1. A hormone that raises the blood calcium level   _____

2. A hormone that lowers the blood glucose level   _____

3. A pancreatic hormone that raises the blood glucose level   _____

4. An adrenal hormone that raises the blood glucose level   _____

5. A hormone that promotes development of secondary sex characteristics   _____

7. DESCRIBE HOW THE HYPOTHALAMUS CONTROLS THE ANTERIOR AND POSTERIOR PITUITARY.

EXERCISE 11-10: The Pituitary Gland (Text Fig. 11-3)

1. Label the parts of the hypothalamo-pituitary system.
2. Color blood vessels red and nerves yellow.

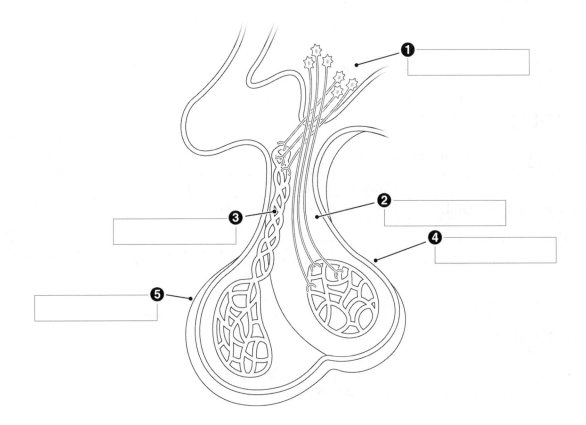

EXERCISE 11-11

Fill in the blank after each statement—does the characteristic apply to the anterior pituitary (AP) or the posterior pituitary (PP)?

1. Secretes hormones synthesized in the hypothalamus _____

2. Consists of neural tissue _____

3. Releases hormones under the regulation of hypothalamic releasing hormones _____

8. LIST TISSUES OTHER THAN THE ENDOCRINE GLANDS THAT PRODUCE HORMONES.

EXERCISE 11-12

Fill in the missing information in the chart below.

Hormone	Site of Synthesis	Effects
Atrial natriuretic peptide		
Thymosin		
	Kidney	Stimulates erythrocyte production

9. LIST SOME MEDICAL USES OF HORMONES.

EXERCISE 11-13

Fill in the column "Medical Uses" in the table prepared for Exercise 11-7 for the following hormones: insulin, cortisol (a glucocorticoid), epinephrine, thyroid hormones, and oxytocin.

10. EXPLAIN HOW THE ENDOCRINE SYSTEM RESPONDS TO STRESS.

EXERCISE 11-14

Explain how the actions of cortisol help an individual cope with a physical stressor such as a predator (or, more realistically, a 5-km road race).

11. REFERRING TO THE CASE STUDY, DISCUSS THE EFFECTS OF INSULIN DEFICIENCY ON BODY FUNCTION.

EXERCISE 11-15

In the list below, circle all of the dysfunctions that would result from insulin deficiency. You should circle one option from each pair.

a. hunger or lack of appetite

b. weight gain or weight loss

c. lethargy or nervousness

d. glucose in the urine or protein in the urine

e. hypoglycemia (low blood glucose concentration) or hyperglycemia (high blood glucose concentration)

12. SHOW HOW WORD PARTS ARE USED TO BUILD WORDS RELATED TO THE ENDOCRINE SYSTEM.

EXERCISE 11-16

Complete the following table by writing the correct word part or meaning in the space provided. Write a word that contains each word part in the Example column.

Word Part	Meaning	Example
1. trop/o	_____	_____
2. _____	cortex	_____
3. -poiesis	_____	_____
4. natri	_____	_____
5. _____	male	_____
6. _____	pancreatic islet, island	_____
7. ren/o	_____	_____
8. -sterone	_____	_____
9. oxy	_____	_____
10. nephr/o	_____	_____

Making the Connections

The following concept map deals with the relationship between the hypothalamus, pituitary gland, and some target organs. Each pair of terms is linked together by a connecting phrase into a sentence. The sentence should be read in the direction of the arrow. Complete the concept map by filling in the appropriate term or phrase. There is one right answer for each term. However, there are many correct answers for the connecting phrases (1, 4, 5, 9, 12).

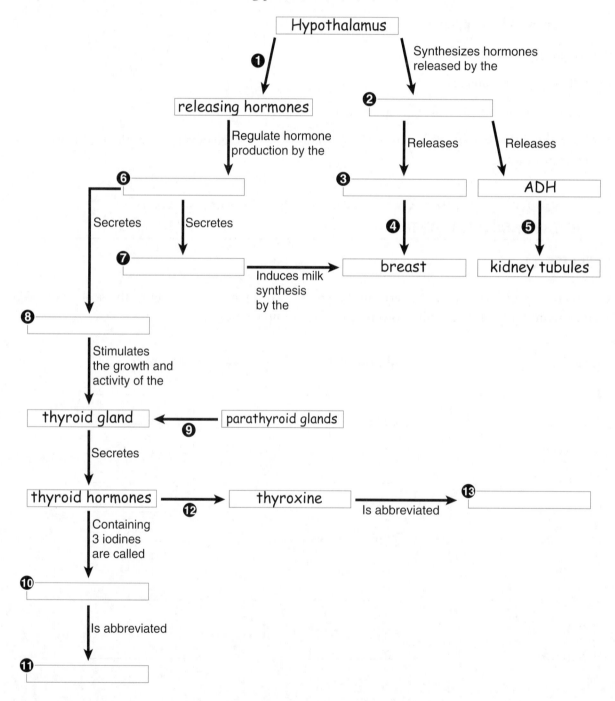

Optional Exercise: Construct your own concept map using the following terms: pancreas, insulin, glucagon, adrenal gland, medulla, cortex, epinephrine, cortisol, aldosterone, raises blood sugar, lowers blood sugar. You can also add other appropriate terms (for instance, target sites or hormone actions).

Testing Your Knowledge

BUILDING UNDERSTANDING

I. MULTIPLE CHOICE

1. Which of these hormones promotes normal growth?
   a. thyroxine/triiodothyronine
   b. cortisol
   c. glucagon
   d. oxytocin

   1. _____

2. What is an androgen?
   a. female sex hormone
   b. glucocorticoid
   c. male sex hormone
   d. atrial hormone

   2. _____

3. Which of the following hormones is NOT produced by the thyroid gland?
   a. calcitonin
   b. thyroxine
   c. triiodothyronine
   d. thyroid-stimulating hormone

   3. _____

4. Which of these hormones causes milk ejection from the breasts?
   a. oxytocin
   b. prolactin
   c. progesterone
   d. estrogen

   4. _____

5. Which of these hormones decreases blood glucose concentrations?
   a. cortisol
   b. aldosterone
   c. insulin
   d. glucagon

   5. _____

6. Which of these glands releases antidiuretic hormone?
   a. anterior pituitary
   b. posterior pituitary
   c. adrenal
   d. pancreas

   6. _____

7. Which of the following hormones is derived from cholesterol?
   a. progesterone
   b. thyroid hormone
   c. growth hormone
   d. luteinizing hormone

   7. _____

8. Which two hormones mediate the stress response?
   a. growth hormone and insulin
   b. testosterone and oxytocin
   c. parathyroid hormone and insulin
   d. epinephrine and cortisol

   8. _____

9. Which pituitary hormone regulates the activity of the thyroid gland?   9. _____
    a. TSH
    b. GH
    c. ACTH
    d. MSH

10. Which of these organs synthesizes erythropoietin?   10. _____
    a. kidneys
    b. skin
    c. heart
    d. placenta

II. COMPLETION EXERCISE

1. An abnormal increase in production of the hormone epinephrine may result from a tumor of the _____.

2. Releasing hormones are sent from the hypothalamus to the anterior pituitary by way of a special circulatory pathway called a(n) _____.

3. When the blood glucose level decreases below average, the islet cells of the pancreas release less insulin. The result is an increase in blood glucose. This is an example of the regulatory mechanism called _____.

4. The hypothalamus stimulates the anterior pituitary to produce ACTH, which, in turn, stimulates hormone production by the _____.

5. The element needed for the production of thyroxine is _____.

6. Local hormones that have a variety of effects, including the promotion of inflammation and the stimulation of uterine contractions, are the _____.

7. A hormone secreted from the posterior pituitary that is involved in water balance is

_____.

8. The primary target tissue for prolactin is the _____.

UNDERSTANDING CONCEPTS

I. TRUE/FALSE

For each question, write T for true or F for false in the blank to the left of each number. If a statement is false, correct it by replacing the *underlined* term and write the correct statement in the blanks below the question.

_____ 1. A deficiency in <u>insulin</u> results in abnormally high concentrations of blood glucose.

_____

_____ 2. Cortisol and the pancreatic hormone <u>insulin</u> both raise blood sugar levels.

_____

_____ 3. <u>Antidiuretic hormone</u> promotes water retention.

_____

_____ 4. The ovaries and testes produce <u>steroid</u> hormones.

_____

_____ 5. Cortisol is produced by the <u>adrenal cortex.</u>

_____

_____ 6. Islet cells are found in the <u>adrenal gland</u>.

_____

_____ 7. ADH and oxytocin are secreted by the <u>anterior</u> lobe of the pituitary.

_____

_____ 8. Atrial natriuretic peptide (ANP) is produced by the <u>kidneys</u>.

_____

II. PRACTICAL APPLICATIONS

Write the appropriate word or phrase in the space provided.

1. Ms. H, age 8, was brought to the clinic because she had been losing weight, was very thirsty, and urinated frequently. A blood chemistry panel showed an extremely high blood glucose reading of 186 mg/dL as well as other abnormal readings. The physician suspected a deficiency in the pancreatic hormone that promotes cellular glucose uptake. This hormone is called _____.

2. Mr. L, age 42, reported to the hospital emergency room with complaints of shortness of breath and heart palpitations. The initial assessment by the nurse included the following findings: rapid heart rate, nervousness with tremor of the hands, skin warm and flushed, sweating, rapid respiration, and protruding eyes. Laboratory tests revealed abnormally high levels of two related hormones produced by the thyroid gland, namely triiodothyronine and _____.

3. After surgery for his endocrine problem, Mr. L had tetany, or contractions of the muscles of the hands and face. This was caused by the incidental surgical removal of the glands that control the release of calcium into the blood. The glands that maintain adequate blood calcium levels are the _____.

4. Ms. M has just been stung by a bee. She is extremely allergic to bees. Her sister gives her a life-saving injection of an adrenal hormone. This hormone is called _____.

5. Ms. Q was supposed to have her baby ten days ago. Her relatives are anxiously awaiting the birth of her child, so she asks her obstetrician if he can do something to hasten the birth of her child. The obstetrician agrees to induce labor using a hormone called _____.

6. Mr. S is preparing for his final law exams and is feeling very stressed. His partner is studying for a physiology exam and mentions that he probably has elevated levels of an anterior pituitary hormone that acts on the adrenal cortex. This hormone is called _____.

7. Ms. J, age 35, is preparing for a weight-lifting competition. She wants to build muscle tissue very rapidly, so a friend recommends that she tries injections of a male steroid known to stimulate tissue building. This steroid is normally produced by the _____.

III. SHORT ESSAYS

1. Explain why hormones, although they circulate throughout the body, exercise their effects only on specific target cells.

   _____

   _____

   _____

2. List two differences between the endocrine system and the nervous system.

   _____

   _____

   _____

3. Name three organs other than endocrine glands that produce hormones, and name a hormone produced in each organ.

   _____

   _____

   _____

4. Compare the anterior and the posterior lobes of the pituitary.

   _____

   _____

   _____

CONCEPTUAL THINKING

1. Mr. J was taking testosterone supplements for many years to build up his muscles. He recently stopped taking the supplements, and a blood test revealed that his blood testosterone concentration was extremely low. Based on your knowledge of negative feedback, can you tell Mr. J. what happened?

   _____

   _____

   _____

2. Young Ms. K suffers from asthma. She uses an inhaler containing epinephrine to treat her attacks. However, lately she has been suffering from a very rapid heartbeat. Her physician advises her to use her inhaler less frequently. Why?

   _____

   _____

   _____

Expanding Your Horizons

In the past, hormones were not available for therapeutic use or were obtained only from cadavers. As you can imagine, hormone supplies were very limited and reserved for cases of hormone deficiency. But many hormones now can be produced in unlimited quantities in the laboratory. This widespread availability has led to abuse by athletes and others trying to gain a competitive advantage. Read about all of the hormones—and other substances—that are banned by the World Anti-Doping Agency (WADA) at the website listed below. You can also access the articles online to read more about the "arms race" between some unscrupulous athletes and the authorities.

- Catlin DH, Fitch KD, Ljungqvist A. Medicine and science in the fight against doping in sport. J Intern Med 2008;264(2):99–114. PMID 18702750. Available at: http://onlinelibrary.wiley.com/doi/10.1111/j.1365-2796.2008.01993.x/pdf
- Saugy M, Robinson N, Saudan C, et al. Human growth hormone doping in sport. Br J Sports Med 2006;40(Suppl 1): i35–i39. PMCID PMC2657499. Available at: http://www.ncbi.nlm.nih.gov/pmc/articles/PMC2657499/
- World Anti Doping Agency Web site. Available at: http://www.wada-ama.org/

Circulation and Body Defense

CHAPTER 12

The Blood

Overview

The blood maintains the constancy of the internal environment through its functions of transportation, regulation, and protection. Blood is composed of two portions: the liquid portion, or plasma, and the formed elements, consisting of cells and cell fragments. The plasma is 91% water and 9% solutes, including proteins, carbohydrates, lipids, electrolytes, and waste products. The formed elements are composed of the erythrocytes, which carry oxygen to the tissues; the leukocytes, which defend the body against invaders; and the platelets, which help prevent blood loss. The forerunners of the blood cells are called hematopoietic stem cells. These are formed in the red bone marrow, where they then develop into the various types of blood cells.

Hemostasis (the prevention of blood loss) is a series of protective mechanisms that occur when a blood vessel is ruptured by an injury. The steps in hemostasis include constriction of the blood vessels, formation of a platelet plug, and formation of a clot (coagulation), a complex series of reactions involving many different factors.

If the quantity of blood in the body is severely reduced because of hemorrhage or disease, the cells suffer from lack of oxygen and nutrients. In such instances, a transfusion may be given after typing and matching the blood of the donor with that of the recipient. Donor red cells with different surface antigens (proteins) than the recipient's red cells will react with antibodies in the recipient's blood plasma, causing harmful agglutination reactions and destruction of the donated cells. Blood is most commonly tested for the ABO system involving antigens A and B. Blood can be packaged and stored in blood banks for use when transfusions are needed. Whenever possible, blood components such as cells, plasma, plasma fractions, or platelets are used. This practice is more efficient and can reduce the chances of incompatibility and transmission of disease.

The Rh factor, another red blood cell protein, also is important in transfusions. If blood containing the Rh factor (Rh positive) is given to a person whose blood lacks that factor (Rh negative), the recipient will produce antibodies to the foreign Rh factor. If an Rh-negative mother is thus sensitized by an Rh-positive fetus, her antibodies may damage fetal red cells in a later pregnancy, resulting in hemolytic disease of the newborn (erythroblastosis fetalis).

Scientists have devised numerous studies to measure the composition of blood. These include the hematocrit, hemoglobin measurements, cell counts, blood chemistry tests, and coagulation studies. Modern laboratories are equipped with automated counters, which rapidly and accurately count blood cells, and with automated analyzers, which measure enzymes, electrolytes, and other constituents of blood serum.

Addressing the Learning Outcomes

1. LIST THE FUNCTIONS OF THE BLOOD.

EXERCISE 12-1

List three functions of blood, and provide an example for each.

1. _____

2. _____

3. _____

2. IDENTIFY THE MAIN COMPONENTS OF PLASMA.

EXERCISE 12-2

Which of the following substances are found in plasma? Circle all that apply.

a. erythrocytes

b. water

c. proteins

d. platelets

e. nutrients

f. electrolytes

3. DESCRIBE THE FORMATION OF BLOOD CELLS.

EXERCISE 12-3

Name the type of stem cell that can develop into all types of blood cells.

_____

4. NAME AND DESCRIBE THE THREE TYPES OF FORMED ELEMENTS IN THE BLOOD AND GIVE THE FUNCTION OF EACH.

EXERCISE 12-4: Composition of Whole Blood (Text Fig. 12-1)

1. Write the names of the different blood components on the appropriate numbered lines in different colors. Use the color red for parts 1, 2, and 3.
2. Color the blood components on the diagram with the appropriate color.

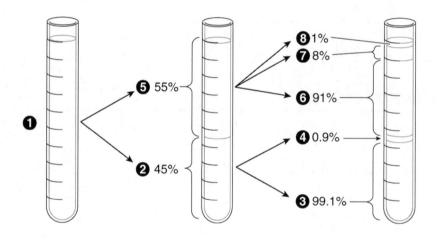

1. _____

2. _____

3. _____

4. _____

5. _____

6. _____

7. _____

8. _____

5. CHARACTERIZE THE FIVE TYPES OF LEUKOCYTES.

EXERCISE 12-5: Leukocytes (Table 12-2)

1. Write the names of the five types of leukocytes on lines 1 to 5.
2. Write the names of the labeled cell parts and other blood cells on lines 6 to 9.

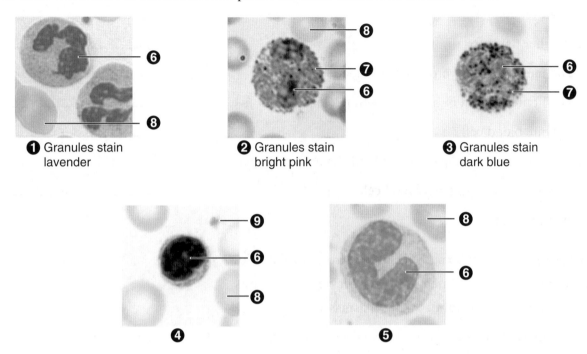

❶ Granules stain lavender

❷ Granules stain bright pink

❸ Granules stain dark blue

❹

❺

1. _____

2. _____

3. _____

4. _____

5. _____

6. _____

7. _____

8. _____

9. _____

EXERCISE 12-6

Write the appropriate term in each blank from the list below.

erythrocyte   platelet   leukocyte   plasma   hemoglobin
albumin   antibodies   complement   serum

1. A red blood cell   _____

2. Another name for thrombocyte   _____

3. The most abundant protein(s) in blood   _____

4. The liquid portion of blood, including clotting factors   _____

5. A white blood cell   _____

6. Enzymes that participate in the battle against pathogens   _____

7. The protein that fills red blood cells   _____

EXERCISE 12-7

Write the appropriate term in each blank from the list below.

neutrophil   macrophage   monocyte   pus
eosinophil   basophil   plasma cell

1. The most abundant type of white blood cell in whole blood   _____

2. A tissue cell that develops from monocytes   _____

3. A lymphocyte that produces antibodies   _____

4. A leukocyte that stains with acidic dyes   _____

5. The largest blood leukocyte   _____

6. A substance that often accumulates when leukocytes are
   actively destroying bacteria   _____

6. DEFINE *HEMOSTASIS* AND CITE THREE STEPS IN HEMOSTASIS.

Also see Exercise 12-9.

EXERCISE 12-8

What is the difference between hemostasis and homeostasis?

_____

_____

_____

7. BRIEFLY DESCRIBE THE STEPS IN BLOOD CLOTTING.

EXERCISE 12-9

Write the appropriate term in each blank from the list below.

vasoconstriction	coagulation	hemorrhage	platelet plug
plasma	serum	thrombin	fibrin
calcium			

1. A collection of cell fragments that temporarily repairs a vessel injury   _____

2. The process of blood clot formation   _____

3. Contraction of smooth muscles in the blood vessel wall   _____

4. Another term for profuse bleeding   _____

5. The active enzyme that converts fibrinogen into fibrin   _____

6. The solid threads that form a blood clot   _____

7. A clotting factor that also is needed to form bone tissue   _____

8. The liquid portion of blood, minus clotting factors   _____

EXERCISE 12-10: Formation of a Blood Clot (Text Fig. 12-7)

Write the correct term in each of the numbered boxes.

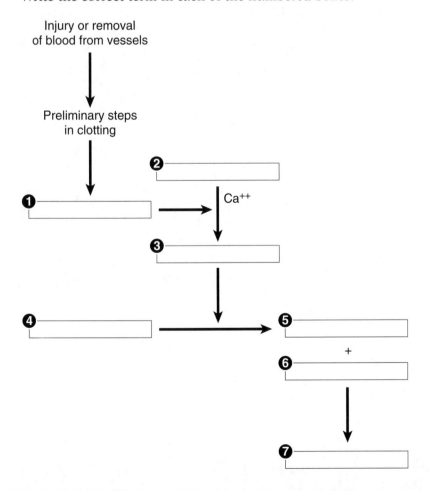

8. DEFINE *BLOOD TYPE* AND EXPLAIN THE RELATION BETWEEN BLOOD TYPE AND TRANSFUSIONS.

EXERCISE 12-11: Blood Typing (Text Fig. 12-8)

Based on the agglutination reactions, write the name of each blood type on the numbered lines.

1. _____

2. _____

3. _____

4. _____

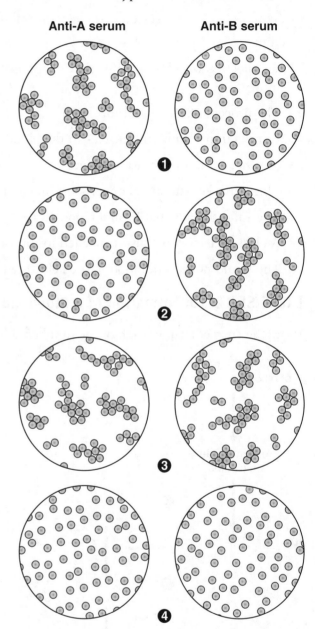

9. EXPLAIN THE BASIS OF Rh INCOMPATIBILITY AND ITS POSSIBLE CONSEQUENCES.

See Exercise 12-12.

10. LIST THE POSSIBLE REASONS FOR TRANSFUSIONS OF WHOLE BLOOD AND BLOOD COMPONENTS.

EXERCISE 12-12

Write the appropriate term in each blank from the list below.

hematocrit   Rh factor   autologous   AB antigen   agglutination

hemapheresis plasmapheresis transfusion antigen

1. The blood antigen involved in hemolytic disease of the newborn, which results from a blood incompatibility between a mother and fetus _____

2. The procedure for removing plasma and returning formed elements to the donor _____

3. The procedure for removing specific components and returning the remainder of the blood to the donor _____

4. Blood donated by an individual for use by the same individual _____

5. The volume percentage of red cells in whole blood _____

6. The administration of blood or blood components from one person to another person _____

7. A general term describing any protein on blood cells that causes incompatibility reactions _____

8. The process by which cells become clumped when mixed with a specific antiserum _____

11. IDENTIFY SIX TYPES OF TESTS USED TO STUDY BLOOD.

EXERCISE 12-13

Which blood test would you use in each situation? Choose the appropriate test from the list below. Each test can be used only once.

red cell count   coagulation study   bone marrow biopsy   blood smear

platelet count

1. Diagnose a clotting deficiency _____

2. Diagnose polycythemia _____

3. Determine the abundance of small cell fragments involved in hemostasis _____

4. A sternal puncture is an example of this type of test _____

5. Count the number of reticulocytes _____

12. REFERRING TO THE CASE STUDY, DESCRIBE THE GENETIC BASIS AND POTENTIAL COMPLICATIONS OF SICKLE CELL ANEMIA.

EXERCISE 12-14

Fill in the blanks in the paragraph below, using the terms from the list below. You will not use all of the terms. Try to complete this exercise without consulting your textbook.

antigens   antibodies   erythrocytes   leukocytes   type B   type AB

agglutination blood smear leucopenia   hematocrit   sickle cell anemia   hemoglobin

oxygen   capillaries   macrophages neutrophils

As part of the normal newborn screening procedures, Cole's blood was subjected to many routine tests. His red blood cells, known as (1) _____, clumped together in the presence of anti-B antiserum but not anti-A antiserum. Thus, (2) _____ in the membranes of his blood cells formed complexes with (3) _____ in the antiserum, a process known as (4) _____. Based on this test, Cole's blood type is (5) _____. Other tests revealed that the major protein in Cole's red blood cells, known as (6) _____, was abnormal. This protein normally transports (7) _____, a gas required for energy generation by cells. When a sample of his blood was examined under a microscope, a procedure known as a (8) _____, abnormally shaped cells were observed. Because of their sickled shape, they tend to block the smallest blood vessels, known as (9) _____. Also, large, monocyte-derived phagocytic cells called (10) _____ tend to destroy the abnormal red blood cells. As a result, the volume percentage of red blood cells in Cole's blood, a measure known as the (11) _____, is abnormally low. This low value indicates that Cole has a disorder called (12) _____.

13. SHOW HOW WORD PARTS ARE USED TO BUILD WORDS RELATED TO THE BLOOD.

EXERCISE 12-15

Complete the following table by writing the correct word part or meaning in the space provided. Write a word that contains each word part in the Example column.

Word Part	Meaning	Example
1. erythr/o	_____	_____
2. _____	blood clot	_____
3. pro-	_____	_____
4. morph/o	_____	_____
5. _____	white, colorless	_____
6. _____	producing, originating	_____
7. hemat/o	_____	_____
8. _____	lack of	_____
9. -emia	_____	_____
10. _____	dissolving	_____

Making the Connections

The following concept map deals with the classification of blood cells. Each pair of terms is linked together by a connecting phrase into a sentence. The sentence should be read in the direction of the arrow. Complete the concept map by filling in the appropriate term or phrase. There is one right answer for each term. However, there are many correct answers for the connecting phrases (5, 6, 8, 10, 12, 14, and 16).

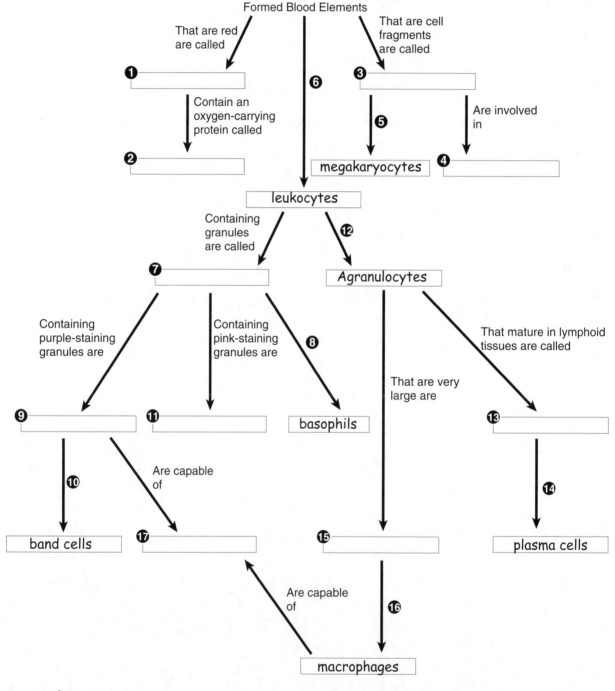

Optional Exercise: Construct your own concept map using the following terms and any others you would like to include: procoagulants, anticoagulants, platelet plug, hemostasis, vasoconstriction, blood clot, fibrinogen, fibrin, prothrombinase, thrombin, serum.

Testing Your Knowledge

BUILDING UNDERSTANDING

I. MULTIPLE CHOICE

1. Plasma can be given to anyone without danger of incompatibility
   because it lacks which of the following substances?   1. _____
   - a. serum
   - b. red cells
   - c. protein
   - d. clotting factors
2. Which blood cell type is also called a polymorph, PMN, or seg?   2. _____
   - a. monocyte
   - b. neutrophil
   - c. basophil
   - d. lymphocyte
3. Which of the following is NOT a type of white blood cell?   3. _____
   - a. thrombocyte
   - b. lymphocyte
   - c. eosinophil
   - d. monocyte
4. Which of these proteins is the enzyme that activates fibrinogen?   4. _____
   - a. albumin
   - b. thrombin
   - c. thromboplastin
   - d. fibrin
5. Which of the following might result in an Rh incompatibility problem?   5. _____
   - a. an Rh-positive mother and an Rh-negative fetus
   - b. an Rh-negative mother and an Rh-positive fetus
   - c. an Rh-negative mother and a type AB fetus
   - d. an Rh-positive mother and an Rh-negative father
6. What is the most abundant protein in plasma?   6. _____
   - a. platelets
   - b. antibodies
   - c. hemoglobin
   - d. albumin
7. Which cell type develops from monocytes?   7. _____
   - a. neutrophils
   - b. macrophages
   - c. plasma cells
   - d. lymphocytes
8. Which antibody classes are present in type B blood?   8. _____
   - a. A
   - b. B
   - c. both A and B
   - d. neither A nor B

9. Which of the following cells is NOT a granulocyte?   9. _____
   a. monocyte
   b. eosinophil
   c. neutrophil
   d. polymorph

II. COMPLETION EXERCISE

1. The volume percentage of red cells in whole blood is the _____.

2. Serious bleeding problems may result from a deficiency of small cell fragments called _____.

3. The gas that is necessary for life and that is transported to all parts of the body by the blood is _____.

4. Some monocytes enter the tissues, mature, and become active phagocytes. These cells are called _____.

5. One waste product of body metabolism is carried to the lungs to be exhaled. This gas is _____.

6. The hormone that stimulates red blood cell production is _____.

7. Blood cells are formed in the _____.

8. The most important function of certain lymphocytes is to engulf disease-producing organisms by the process of _____.

9. The inorganic chemical element that characterizes hemoglobin is _____.

UNDERSTANDING CONCEPTS

I. TRUE/FALSE

For each question, write T for true or F for false in the blank to the left of each number. If a statement is false, correct it by replacing the <u>underlined</u> term and write the correct statement in the blanks below the question.

_____ 1. Eosinophils and basophils are <u>granular</u> leukocytes.

_____

_____ 2. If the formed elements are returned to the blood donor, the procedure is called <u>plasmapheresis</u>.

_____

_____ 3. A microliter (mcl) of blood contains about 5 million <u>leukocytes</u>.

_____

_____ 4. The hormone that stimulates red blood cell production is produced by the <u>kidneys</u>.

_____

_____ 5. <u>Type AB</u> blood contains antibodies to both A and B antigens.

_____

_____ 6. Platelets are fragments of large cells called <u>agranulocytes</u>.

_____

_____ 7. Substances that induce blood clotting are called <u>procoagulants</u>.

_____

_____ 8. The watery fluid that remains after a blood clot has been removed from the blood is
<u>plasma</u>.

_____

II. PRACTICAL APPLICATIONS

Study each discussion. Then write the appropriate word or phrase in the space provided.

➤ Group A

1. A young girl named AL fell off her bike, sustaining a deep gash to her leg that bled copiously
   from a severed vessel. In describing this type of bleeding, the doctor in the emergency clinic
   used the word _____.

2. While the physician attended to the wound, the technician drew blood for typing and other
   studies. AL's blood did not agglutinate with either anti-A or anti-B serum. Her blood was
   classified as type _____.

3. Young AL required a blood transfusion. The only type of blood she could receive is type
   _____.

4. Further testing of AL's blood revealed that it lacked the Rh factor. She was, therefore, said to
   be _____.

5. If AL were to be given a transfusion of Rh-positive blood, she might become sensitized to
   the Rh protein. In that event, her blood would produce counteracting substances called
   _____.

6. The technician examined AL's blood under the microscope and noticed some red
   blood cells were shaped like crescent-moons. AL may have the disorder called
   _____.

➤ Group B

1. Mr. KK, age 72, had an injury riding his motorized scooter down a steep hill. He suffered only minor scrapes, but he came to the hospital because his scrapes did not stop bleeding. The three-step process by which blood loss is prevented or minimized is called _____.

2. The physician discovered that Mr. KK was the great-great-great grandson of Queen Victoria. Like many of her offspring, Mr. KK suffers from a deficiency of a clotting factor. Clotting factors participate in the stage of hemostasis known as _____.

3. Mr. KK must be treated with a rich source of clotting factors. The doctor gets a bag of frozen plasma, which has a white powdery substance at the bottom of the bag. The substance is called _____.

4. Mr. KK also mentions that he has been very tired and pale lately. His cook recently retired, and he has been surviving on dill pickles and crackers. The physician suspects a deficiency in an element required to synthesize hemoglobin. This element is called _____.

5. The physician orders a test to determine the proportion of red blood cells in his blood. The result of this test is called the _____.

6. The test confirms that Mr. KK does not have enough red blood cells, due to a dietary deficiency. This deficiency impairs the ability of his blood to carry the gas known as _____.

➤ Group C

1. Ms. J, an elite cyclist, has come to the hospital complaining of a pounding headache. The physician, Dr. L, takes a sample of her blood, and notices that it is very thick. He decides to count her red blood cells, but the automatic cell counter is broken. Dr. L calls for a technician to perform a visual count using the microscope and a special slide called a(n) _____.

2. The technician comes back with a result of 7.5 million cells/mL. This count is abnormally high, suggesting a diagnosis of _____.

3. Dr. L is immediately suspicious. He asks Ms. J if she consumes any performance-enhancing drugs. Ms. J admits that she has been taking a hormone to increase red blood cell synthesis. This hormone is called _____.

4. Dr. L tells Ms. J that she is at risk for blood clot formation. He tells her to stop taking the hormone and to take aspirin for a few days to inhibit blood clotting. Drugs that inhibit clotting are called _____.

III. SHORT ESSAYS

1. What kind of information can be obtained from blood chemistry tests?

_____

_____

_____

_____

_____

2. Briefly describe the final events in blood clot formation, naming the substances involved in each step.

_____

_____

_____

_____

_____

3. Name one reason to transfuse an individual with:

a. whole blood

_____

b. platelets

_____

c. plasma

_____

d. plasma protein

_____

CONCEPTUAL THINKING

1. A dehydrated individual will have an elevated hematocrit. Explain why.

   _____

   _____

   _____

2. Mr. R needs a blood transfusion. He has type AB blood. The doctor is considering a transfusion using A blood.

   a. Which antigens are present on his blood cells?

   _____

   b. Which antibodies will be present in his blood?

   _____

   c. Which antigens will be present on donor blood cells?

   _____

   d. Is this blood transfusion safe? Why or why not?

   _____

Expanding Your Horizons

Have you ever watched vampire shows, such as the *Twilight* series or *True Blood?* Imagine how much easier life would be for vampires if they could buy blood in the grocery stores. And, in our vampire-free world, a safe, effective artificial blood substitute would save dollars and lives. These substitutes would be free of the problems associated with normal blood transfusions: contamination with HIV or hepatitis, incompatibility reactions, short shelf life, stringent storage conditions, and limited supply. Billions of dollars have gone into the search for artificial blood, and some compounds have been used when blood supplies run short. However, none of the currently available substitutes are safe—they all appear to increase the risk of heart attack. You can read more about the search for a safe blood substitute on the Web sites below, or do a search for "artificial blood."

- Davis R. Study: Blood substitute increases risk of death. USA Today 4/28/2008. Available at: http://www.usatoday.com/news/health/2008-04-28-fake-blood-risks_N.htm
- http://web.me.com/profchriscooper/Home/

CHAPTER

13

The Heart

Overview

The ceaseless beat of the heart day and night throughout one's entire lifetime is such an obvious key to the presence of life that it is no surprise that this organ has been the subject of wonderment and poetry. When the heart stops pumping, life ceases. The cells must have oxygen, and it is the heart's pumping action that propels oxygen-rich blood to them.

In size, the heart is roughly the size of one's fist. It is located between the lungs, more than half to the left of the midline, with the **apex** (point) directed toward the left. Below is the **diaphragm**, the dome-shaped muscle that separates the thoracic cavity from the abdominopelvic cavity.

The heart consists of two sides separated by septa. The septa keep blood that is higher in oxygen entirely separate from blood that is lower in oxygen. The two sides pump in unison, the right side pumping blood to the lungs to be pick up more oxygen and drop off carbon dioxide, and the left side pumping blood to all other parts of the body.

Each side of the heart is divided into two parts or **chambers**. The upper chamber or **atrium** on each side is the receiving chamber for blood returning to the heart. The lower chamber or **ventricle** is the strong pumping chamber. Because the ventricles pump more forcefully, their walls are thicker than the walls of the atria. **Valves** between the chambers keep the blood flowing forward as the heart pumps. The muscle of the heart wall, the **myocardium**, has special features to enhance its pumping efficiency. The coronary circulation supplies blood directly to the myocardium.

The heartbeat originates within the heart at the **sinoatrial (SA) node**, often called the pacemaker. Electrical impulses from the pacemaker spread through special conducting fibers in the wall of the heart to induce contractions, first of the two atria and then of the two ventricles. While the atria contract the ventricles relax, and vice versa. After ventricular contraction finishes, the entire heart relaxes and fills with blood. For each heart chamber, the relaxation phase is called **diastole**, and the contraction phase is called **systole**. One **cardiac cycle** includes all of the events of a single heartbeat, that is, atrial systole, ventricular systole, and then diastole of all heart chambers. The heart rate is influenced by the nervous system and other circulating factors, such as hormones and drugs.

Addressing the Learning Outcomes

1. DESCRIBE THE THREE TISSUE LAYERS OF THE HEART WALL.

See Exercises 13-1, 13-2, and 13-3.

2. DESCRIBE THE LOCATION AND STRUCTURE OF THE PERICARDIUM AND CITE ITS FUNCTIONS.

EXERCISE 13-1: Layers of the Heart Wall and Pericardium (Text Fig. 13-2)

1. Write the terms *heart wall* and *serous pericardium* in the appropriate boxes.
2. Write the names of structures 3 through 8 on the numbered lines in different colors. Use black for structure 6, because it will not be colored.
3. Color the structures on the diagram (except structure 6) with the appropriate colors.

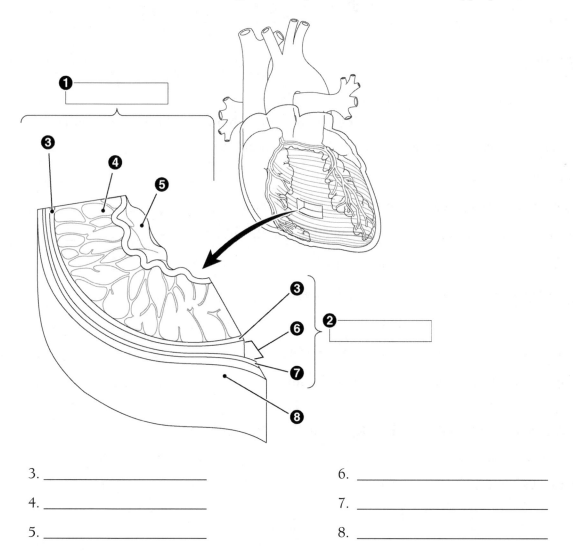

3. _____   6. _____

4. _____   7. _____

5. _____   8. _____

EXERCISE 13-2

Fill in the blanks of the concept map below.

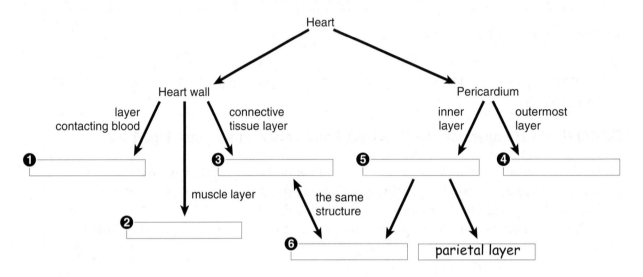

EXERCISE 13-3

Write the appropriate term in each blank from the list below.

base   apex   endocardium   epicardium   fibrous pericardium

myocardium   serous pericardium   visceral layer   parietal layer

1. The pointed, inferior portion of the heart   _____

2. The membrane consisting of a visceral and a parietal layer   _____

3. A layer of epithelial cells in contact with blood within the heart   _____

4. The heart layer containing intercalated disks   _____

5. The outermost layer of the sac enclosing the heart   _____

6. An alternate term for the epicardium   _____

7. The site where the major vessels attach to the heart   _____

8. The heart wall layer composed of connective tissue   _____

3. COMPARE THE FUNCTIONS OF THE RIGHT AND LEFT CHAMBERS OF THE HEART.

See Exercises 13-4 and 13-5.

4. NAME THE VALVES AT THE ENTRANCE AND EXIT OF EACH VENTRICLE AND IDENTIFY THE FUNCTION OF EACH.

EXERCISE 13-4: The Heart and Great Vessels (Text Fig. 13-4)

1. Label the indicated parts. Hint: Structures 5 and 14 are chambers.
2. Use arrows to show the direction of blood flow. If you like, use red arrows for blood high in oxygen and blue arrows for blood low in oxygen.

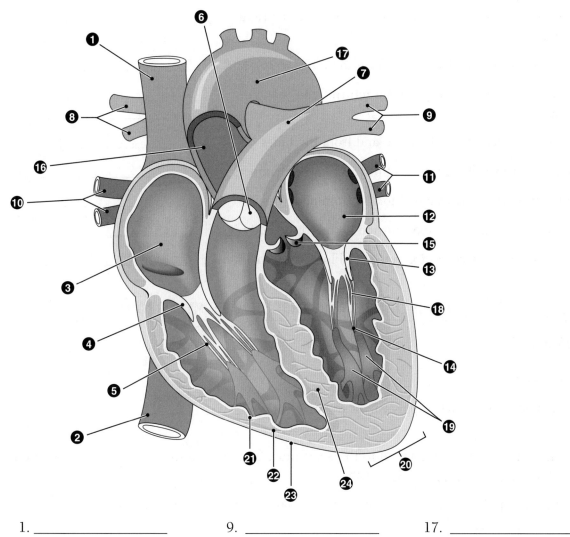

1. _____	9. _____	17. _____
2. _____	10. _____	18. _____
3. _____	11. _____	19. _____
4. _____	12. _____	20. _____
5. _____	13. _____	21. _____
6. _____	14. _____	22. _____
7. _____	15. _____	23. _____
8. _____	16. _____	24. _____

EXERCISE 13-5

Write the appropriate term in each blank from the list below.

left ventricle   right ventricle   left atrium   right atrium

atrioventricular valve   pulmonary valve   pulmonary circuit   aortic valve

systemic circuit

1. The chamber that pumps blood to the lungs   _____

2. The valve that prevents blood from returning to the right
   ventricle   _____

3. The chamber that receives blood from the lungs   _____

4. The valve that prevents blood from returning to the left
   ventricle   _____

5. The pathway that carries blood to and from the lungs   _____

6. One of two valves dividing the upper and lower chambers   _____

7. The pathway that carries blood to and from body tissues   _____

8. The chamber that pumps oxygen-rich blood to the body   _____

9. The chamber that receives oxygen-poor blood from the body   _____

5. BRIEFLY DESCRIBE BLOOD CIRCULATION THROUGH THE MYOCARDIUM.

EXERCISE 13-6

Fill in the blanks.

1. All the blood vessels that supply the heart constitute the _____
   circulation.

2. The main arteries supplying blood to the heart muscle branch off from the aorta just superior
   to the _____ valve.

3. Blood from capillaries in the heart muscle eventually enters a dilated vein called the
   _____.

4. Blood from the heart muscle eventually drains into the _____ atrium.

6. BRIEFLY DESCRIBE THE CARDIAC CYCLE.

EXERCISE 13-7

Fill in the blank after each event—does it occur in complete diastole (D), atrial systole (A), or ventricular systole (V)?

1. The ventricles are contracting _____

2. The atria are contracting _____

3. Blood is entering the aorta _____

4. Neither the ventricles nor the atria are contracting _____

5. The atrioventricular valves are closed _____

EXERCISE 13-8

Write the appropriate term in each blank from the list below.

diastole   atrial systole   ventricular systole   cardiac output   stroke volume

1. The amount of blood ejected from a ventricle with each beat   _____

2. The stage of the cardiac cycle that directly follows the resting period _____

3. The stage of the cardiac cycle that precedes the resting period   _____

4. The volume of blood pumped by each ventricle in 1 minute   _____

5. The resting period of the cardiac cycle   _____

7. NAME AND LOCATE THE COMPONENTS OF THE HEART'S CONDUCTION SYSTEM.

EXERCISE 13-9: The Conduction System of the Heart (Text Fig. 13-9)

1. Label the heart chambers (bullets 1 to 4).
2. Label the parts of the conducting system (bullets 5 to 10). Draw arrows to indicate the direction of impulse conduction.

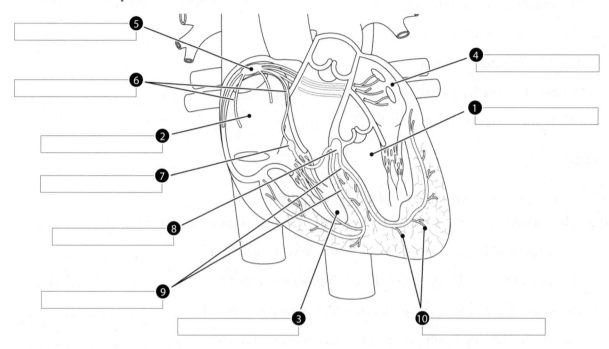

EXERCISE 13-10

Write the appropriate term in each blank from the list below.

atrioventricular bundle	Purkinje fibers	sinus rhythm
sinoatrial node	atrioventricular node	internodal pathways

1. The group of conduction fibers found in the ventricles' walls _____

2. The mass of conduction tissue located in the septum at the bottom of the right atrium _____

3. A normal heart beat, originating from the normal heart pacemaker _____

4. The group of conduction fibers carrying impulses from the AV node _____

5. The name of the normal heart pacemaker, located in the upper wall of the right atrium _____

8. EXPLAIN THE EFFECTS OF THE AUTONOMIC NERVOUS SYSTEM (ANS) ON THE HEART RATE.

EXERCISE 13-11

Fill in the blank after each statement—does the characteristic refer to the parasympathetic nervous system (P) or the sympathetic nervous system (S)?

1. Regulates heart activity via the vagus nerve _____

2. Uses ganglia located close to the spinal cord _____

3. Decreases the heart rate _____

4. Increases the force of each contraction _____

5. Increases the heart rate _____

9. LIST AND DEFINE SEVERAL TERMS THAT DESCRIBE VARIATIONS IN HEART RATES.

EXERCISE 13-12

Write the appropriate term in each blank from the list below.
bradycardia   tachycardia   sinus arrhythmia   extrasystole

1. A beat that comes before the normal beat _____

2. A normal variation in heart rate caused by changes in breathing rate _____

3. A heart rate of less than 60 beats/min _____

4. A heart rate of greater than 100 beats/min _____

10. EXPLAIN WHAT PRODUCES EACH OF THE TWO NORMAL HEART SOUNDS AND IDENTIFY THE USUAL CAUSE OF A MURMUR.

EXERCISE 13-13

Fill in the blanks.

1. The "lub" sound is caused by the closure of the _____ valves.

2. The "dub" sound is caused by the closure of the _____ valves.

3. An abnormal sound caused by a structural problem in the heart or nearby vessels is called a(n) _____ murmur.

4. A sound heard during the workings of a healthy heart is called a(n) _____ murmur.

11. DESCRIBE SEVERAL LIFESTYLE CHOICES THAT CAN HELP MAINTAIN HEART HEALTH.

EXERCISE 13-14

Label each of the following statements as true (T) or false (F). The risk of heart disease is increased if you:

1. Smoke _____

2. Have low blood pressure _____

3. Have diabetes mellitus _____

4. Exercise regularly _____

5. Are a 30-year-old male (compared to a 30-year-old female) _____

6. Tend to deposit fat on the thighs (rather than around the abdomen) _____

7. Eat more unsaturated fat and relatively little saturated fat _____

12. BRIEFLY DESCRIBE METHODS USED TO STUDY THE HEART.

EXERCISE 13-15

Write the appropriate term in each blank from the list below.

stethoscope   echocardiography   catheterization   homocysteine

coronary angiography   electrocardiography   C-reactive protein

1. Technique that uses ultrasound to study the heart as it beats _____

2. A marker of inflammation that can predict heart attack risk _____

3. Technique that measures the electrical activity of the heart _____

4. Instrument used to detect heart murmurs by their sound _____

5. Any procedure in which an extremely thin tube is inserted into a vessel _____

6. A procedure that uses a catheter and dyes to visualize the heart's blood vessels _____

13. REFERRING TO THE CASE STUDY, LIST THE EMERGENCY AND SURGICAL PROCEDURES COMMONLY PERFORMED FOLLOWING A MYOCARDIAL INFARCTION AND EXPLAIN WHY THEY ARE DONE.

EXERCISE 13-16

In the lines below, list three emergency measures, three administered medications, and one surgical measure that Jim (the case study patient) received. Briefly describe the purpose of each.
Emergency measures:

1. _____

2. _____

3. _____

Medications:

1. _____

2. _____

3. _____

Surgery:

1. _____

14. SHOW HOW WORD PARTS ARE USED TO BUILD WORDS RELATED TO THE HEART.

EXERCISE 13-17

Complete the following table by writing the correct word part or meaning in the space provided. Write a word that contains each word part in the Example column.

Word Part	Meaning	Example
1. _____	chest	_____
2. sin/o	_____	_____
3. _____	vessel	_____
4. cardi/o	_____	_____
5. _____	lung	_____
6. _____	slow	_____
7. _____	rapid	_____

Making the Connections

The following flow chart deals with the passage of blood through the heart. Beginning with the right atrium, outline the structures a blood cell would pass through in the correct order by filling in the boxes. Use the following terms: left atrium, left ventricle, right ventricle, right AV valve, left AV valve, pulmonary semilunar valve, aortic semilunar valve, superior/inferior vena cava, right lung, left lung, aorta, left pulmonary artery, right pulmonary artery, left pulmonary veins, right pulmonary veins, body. You can write the names of structures that encounter blood high in oxygen in red and the names of structures that encounter blood low in oxygen in blue.

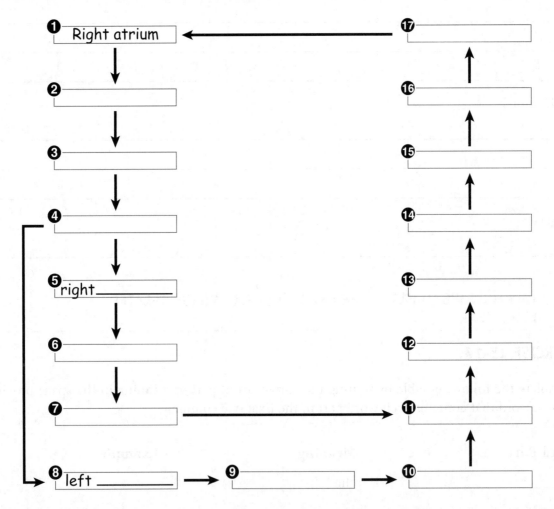

1. Right atrium
2.
3.
4.
5. right
6.
7.
8. left
9.
10.
11.
12.
13.
14.
15.
16.
17.

Optional Exercise: Make your own concept map, based on the events of the cardiac cycle. Choose your own terms to incorporate into your map, or use the following list: AV valves open, AV valves closed, blood flow from atria to ventricles, blood flow from ventricles to arteries, atrial diastole, atrial systole, ventricular diastole, ventricular systole. There will be many links between the different terms.

Testing Your Knowledge

BUILDING UNDERSTANDING

I. MULTIPLE CHOICE

Select the best answer and write the letter of your choice in the blank.

1. How long does it take to complete an average cardiac cycle?
    a. 8 seconds
    b. 5 seconds
    c. 0.8 second
    d. 30 seconds

    1. _____

2. Which of these terms describes the volume of blood pumped by each ventricle in 1 minute?
    a. stroke volume
    b. cardiac output
    c. heart rate
    d. ejection rate

    2. _____

3. Which of the following is NOT a part of the conduction system of the heart?
    a. atrioventricular bundle
    b. atrioventricular valve
    c. Purkinje fibers
    d. atrioventricular node

    3. _____

4. Which of these terms best describes an abnormally high heart rate?
    a. extrasystole
    b. hypocardia
    c. stenosis
    d. tachycardia

    4. _____

5. What is the effect of the parasympathetic nervous system on the heart?
    a. increase heart rate but not myocardial contraction strength
    b. increase heart rate and myocardial contraction strength
    c. decrease heart rate but not myocardial contraction strength
    d. decrease heart rate and myocardial contraction strength

    5. _____

6. Which technique uses ultrasound waves to image the heart in action?
    a. fluoroscopy
    b. echocardiography
    c. electrocardiography
    d. angiography

    6. _____

7. Which vein carries blood from the coronary circulation back into the right atrium?
    a. right coronary artery
    b. interatrial septum
    c. pulmonary vein
    d. coronary sinus

    7. _____

8. Which heart layer is formed of muscle tissue?   8. _____
   a. myocardium
   b. endocardium
   c. epicardium
   d. pericardium

9. Which membranes are separated by the pericardial space?   9. _____
   a. the fibrous pericardium and the serous pericardium
   b. the visceral and parietal layers of the serous pericardium
   c. the epicardium and the pericardium
   d. the myocardium and the epicardium

10. Which heart chamber receives blood from the lungs?   10. _____
   a. right ventricle
   b. left ventricle
   c. right atrium
   d. left atrium

II. COMPLETION EXERCISE

Write the word or phrase that correctly completes each sentence.

1. The autonomic nerve that slows the heart beat is the _____.

2. The sac that surrounds the heart is the _____.

3. An abnormality in the rhythm of the heartbeat is a(n) _____.

4. The valve controlling the flow of blood out of the left ventricle is the
   _____.

5. One complete cycle of heart contraction and relaxation is called the
   _____.

6. The fibrous threads connecting the AV valves to muscles in the heart wall are called
   the _____.

7. The right atrioventricular valve is also known as the _____.

8. Normal heart sounds heard while the heart is working are called _____.

9. The atrioventricular valves are closed during the phase of the cardiac cycle known as
   ventricular _____.

UNDERSTANDING CONCEPTS

I. TRUE/FALSE

For each question, write T for true or F for false in the blank to the left of each number. If a statement is false, correct it by replacing the underlined term and write the correct statement in the blanks below the question.

_____ 1. Heart rate increases in response to parasympathetic stimulation.

_____

_____ 2. The circulatory system of the fetus has certain adaptations for the purpose of bypassing the kidneys.

_____

_____ 3. A heart rate of 150 beats/min is described as tachycardia.

_____

_____ 4. Blood in the heart chambers comes into contact with the epicardium.

_____

_____ 5. The aorta is part of the pulmonary circuit.

_____

_____ 6. Nerve impulses travel down the internodal pathways from the AV node.

_____

_____ 7. A heart rhythm originating at the SA node is termed a sinus rhythm.

_____

II. PRACTICAL APPLICATIONS

Study each discussion. Then write the appropriate word or phrase in the space provided.

➤ Group A

1. Ms. J, age 82, was participating in a lawn bowling tournament when she suddenly collapsed with chest pain. The paramedics were preparing her for transport to the hospital when they noted a sudden onset of pale skin and unconsciousness. The heart monitor showed an extremely rapid heartbeat, known as _____.

2. The paramedics administered an electric shock using an automated defibrillator with the aim of restoring the normal heart rhythm, which is called a(n) _____.

3. In the hospital emergency room, further testing revealed that Ms J had suffered a heart attack. The scientific name for this event is _____.

4. Ms J's symptoms resulted from damage to the middle layer of the heart wall, which is known as the _____.

5. Further testing revealed a blood clot in the blood vessels supplying the heart with blood, collectively known as the _____.

➤ Group B

1. Baby L has just been born. The obstetrician listens to her heartbeat using an instrument called a(n) _____.

2. The doctor notices an abnormality in the second heart sound (or "dup"), which is largely caused by the closure of the two _____.

3. This abnormal sound probably reflects a structural problem with Baby L's heart and is thus termed a(n) _____.

4. The baby is sent for a test that uses ultrasound waves to examine her heart structure. A hole is observed between the two lower chambers of her heart. These chambers are collectively known as the _____.

5. In addition to the two defects already described, a malformation was detected in the major artery carrying oxygen-rich blood from the heart. This artery is known as the _____.

III. SHORT ESSAYS

1. Although the heartbeat originates within the heart itself, it is influenced by factors in the internal environment. Describe some of these factors that can affect the heart.

_____

_____

_____

_____

2. List, in order, all of the vessels, chambers and valves a blood cell will encounter as it enters the heart from the body and then exits the heart heading towards the lungs. Begin with the vessel that drains into the heart, and end with the vessel that receives blood pumped from the heart.

_____

_____

_____

_____

CONCEPTUAL THINKING

1. Atropine is a drug that inhibits activity of the parasympathetic nervous system. Discuss the effects of atropine on the heart. How does the parasympathetic nervous system affect the heart, and which aspects of heart function will be affected and which will be unaffected?

_____

_____

_____

2. Mr. J is undertaking a gentle exercise program, primarily involving walking, to lose weight. His heart rate is 100 beats/min and his stroke volume is 75 mL. What is his cardiac output in liters, and what does cardiac output mean?

_____

_____

_____

_____

Expanding Your Horizons

How low can you go? You may have heard of the exploits of free divers, who dive to tremendous depths without the aid of SCUBA equipment. The world record for assisted free diving is held by Pipin Ferreras, who dove to 170 m (558 ft) with the aid of a sled. Free diving is not without its dangers. Pipin's wife (Audrey) died during a world record attempt. Free diving is facilitated by the dive reflex, which allows mammals to hold their breath for long periods of time underwater. Immersing one's face in cold water induces bradycardia and diverts blood away from the periphery. How would these modifications increase the ability to free dive? You can learn more about the underlying mechanisms, rationale, and dangers of the dive reflex by performing a Web site search for "dive reflex." Information is also available in the article listed below.

- Hurwitz BE, Furedy JJ. The human dive reflex: an experimental, topographical, and physiological analysis. Physiol Behav 1986;36:287–294.

CHAPTER
14

Blood Vessels and Blood Circulation

Overview

The blood vessels are classified as arteries, veins, or capillaries according to their function. **Arteries** carry blood away from the heart, **veins** return blood to the heart, and **capillaries** are the site of gas, nutrient, and waste exchange between the blood and tissues. Small arteries are called **arterioles**, and small veins are called **venules**. The walls of the arteries are thicker and more elastic than the walls of the veins in order to withstand higher pressure. All vessels are lined with a single layer of simple epithelium called **endothelium**. The smallest vessels, the capillaries, are made only of this single layer of cells. The exchange of fluid between capillaries and interstitial spaces is influenced by **blood pressure**, which pushes fluid out of the capillary, and **osmotic pressure**, which draws fluid back in. Blood pressure is regulated over the short term by the **cardiac output** and the **total peripheral resistance**. Long-term changes in overall blood volume and in the length and compliance of the blood vessels also alter blood pressure.

The vessels carry blood through two circuits. The **pulmonary circuit** transports blood between the heart and the lungs for gas exchange. The **systemic circuit** distributes blood high in oxygen to all body tissues and returns the blood low in oxygen to the heart.

The walls of the vessels, especially those of the small arteries, contain smooth muscle that is under the control of the involuntary nervous system. Increased contraction of the muscle narrows the vessel's lumen (opening); relaxation has the opposite effect. By controlling vascular smooth muscle contraction, the autonomic nervous system can modulate blood pressure and blood distribution. Increasing the lumen diameter, a process known as **vasodilation**, reduces blood pressure if it occurs in many blood vessels at once. Vasodilation of a particular blood vessel increases the blood supply to the region supplied by the vessel. **Vasoconstriction**, or decreasing the lumen diameter, has the opposite effects.

Several forces work together to drive blood back to the heart in the venous system. Contraction of skeletal muscles compresses the veins and pushes blood forward, **valves** in the veins keep blood from flowing backward, and changes in intrathoracic pressure that occur during breathing help to drive blood back to the heart. The **pulse rate** and **blood pressure** can provide information about an individual's cardiovascular health.

Addressing the Learning Outcomes

1. DIFFERENTIATE AMONG THE FIVE TYPES OF BLOOD VESSELS WITH REGARD TO STRUCTURE AND FUNCTION.

EXERCISE 14-1: Sections of Small Blood Vessels (Text Fig. 14-2)

1. Write the names of the different vessel types on lines 1 to 5.
2. Write the names of the different vascular layers on the appropriate numbered lines (6–10) in different colors. Use black for structure 10 because it will not be colored.
3. Color the structures on the diagram with the appropriate color (except for structure 10).
4. Draw an arrow in the box to indicate the direction of blood flow.

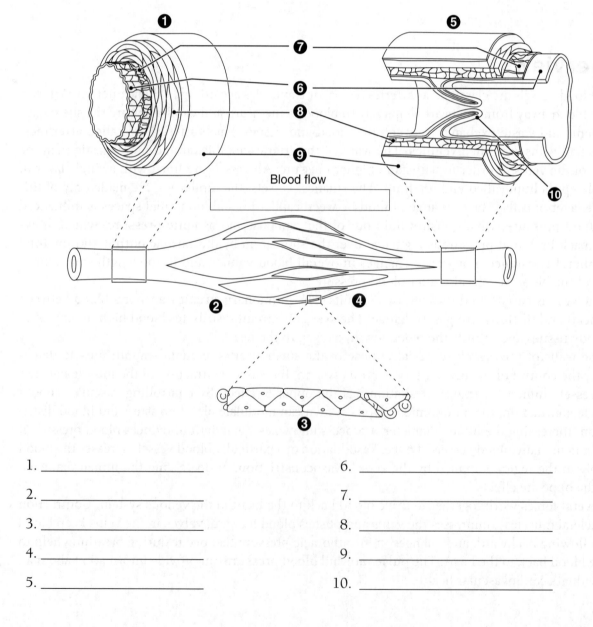

Blood flow

1. _____	6. _____
2. _____	7. _____
3. _____	8. _____
4. _____	9. _____
5. _____	10. _____

EXERCISE 14-2

Write the appropriate term in each blank from the list below.

artery   capillary   vein   venule   arteriole

1. A small vessel through which exchanges between the blood and the cells take place   _____

2. A vessel that receives blood from the capillaries   _____

3. A vessel that branches off the aorta   _____

4. A small vessel that delivers blood to the capillaries   _____

5. A vessel that receives blood from venules and delivers it to the heart   _____

2. COMPARE THE PULMONARY AND SYSTEMIC CIRCUITS RELATIVE TO LOCATION AND FUNCTION.

EXERCISE 14-3: The Cardiovascular System (Text Fig. 14-1)

1. Label the indicated parts.
2. Color the blood high in oxygen red and the blood low in oxygen blue.
3. Use arrows to show the direction of blood flow.
4. Write (P) beside the name of each blood vessel and organ (other than the heart) that is part of the pulmonary circuit.
5. Write (S) beside the name of each blood vessel (other than the heart) that is part of the systemic circuit.

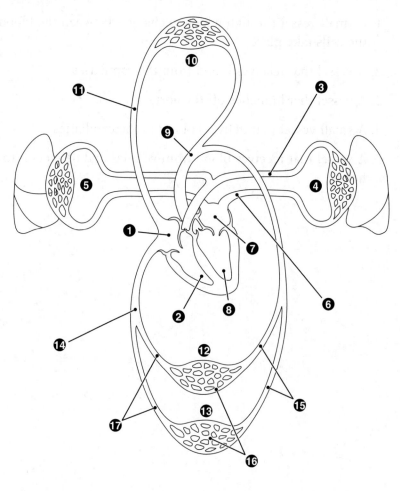

1. _____
2. _____
3. _____
4. _____
5. _____
6. _____
7. _____
8. _____
9. _____
10. _____
11. _____
12. _____
13. _____
14. _____
15. _____
16. _____
17. _____

3. NAME THE FOUR SECTIONS OF THE AORTA AND LIST THE MAIN BRANCHES OF EACH SECTION.

EXERCISE 14-4: Aorta and Its Branches (Text Fig. 14-4)

1. Write the names of the aortic sections on lines 1 to 4 in different colors, and color the appropriate structures on the diagram. Although the aorta is continuous, lines have been added to the diagram to indicate the boundaries of the different sections.
2. Write the names of the aortic branches on the appropriate lines 5 to 22 in different colors, and color the corresponding artery on the diagram. Use the same color for structures 8 and 9 and for structures 7 and 10. Use black for structure 15 because it will not be colored. Color all of the arteries, even if only one is labeled (e.g., bullet 11).

1. _____
2. _____
3. _____
4. _____
5. _____
6. _____
7. _____
8. _____
9. _____
10. _____
11. _____
12. _____
13. _____
14. _____
15. _____
16. _____
17. _____
18. _____
19. _____
20. _____
21. _____
22. _____

4. TRACE THE PATHWAY OF BLOOD THROUGH THE MAIN ARTERIES OF THE UPPER AND LOWER LIMBS.

EXERCISE 14-5: Principal Systemic Arteries (Text Fig. 14-5)

1. Write the names of the principal systemic arteries on the appropriate lines in different, preferably darker, colors. Felt tip pens would work well for this exercise. Use black for structure 14, because it will not be colored.
2. Outline the arteries on the diagram with the appropriate color. If appropriate, color the left and right versions of each artery (for instance, you can color the right and left anterior tibial arteries).

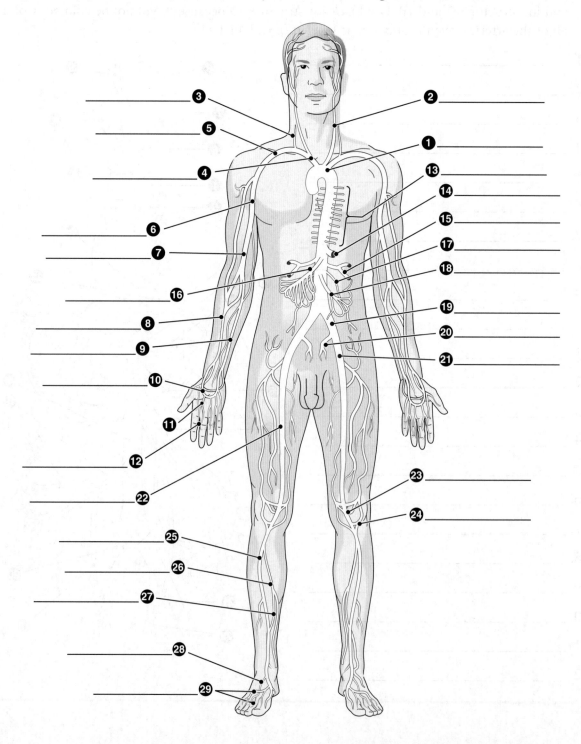

EXERCISE 14-6

Write the appropriate term in each blank from the list below.

coronary arteries   carotid arteries   lumbar arteries   common iliac arteries   phrenic arteries

intercostal arteries   ovarian arteries   renal arteries   suprarenal arteries   brachial arteries

1. Paired branches of the abdominal aorta that supply the diaphragm   _____

2. The vessels that branch off the ascending aorta and supply the heart muscle   _____

3. The large, paired branches of the abdominal aorta that supply blood to the kidneys   _____

4. The vessels formed by final division of the abdominal aorta   _____

5. The vessels that supply the head and neck on each side   _____

6. The paired arteries that branch into the radial and ulnar arteries   _____

7. A group of paired vessels that extend between the ribs   _____

8. Paired branches of the abdominal aorta that extend into the abdominal wall musculature   _____

EXERCISE 14-7

Write the appropriate term in each blank from the list below.

ascending aorta   aortic arch   thoracic aorta   abdominal aorta

brachiocephalic artery   celiac trunk   hepatic artery

1. The short artery that branches into the left gastric artery, the splenic artery, and the hepatic artery   _____

2. A large vessel found within the pericardial sac   _____

3. The portion of the aorta supplying the upper extremities, neck, and head   _____

4. The large vessel that branches into the right subclavian artery and the right common carotid artery   _____

5. The most inferior portion of the aorta   _____

6. The vessel supplying oxygen-rich blood to the liver   _____

5. DEFINE *ANASTOMOSIS*, CITE ITS FUNCTION, AND GIVE SEVERAL EXAMPLES.

EXERCISE 14-8: Principal Systemic Arteries of the Head (Text Fig. 14-6)

1. Write the names of the anastomosis on line 3 in black.
2. Write the names of the arteries on the appropriate lines in different, preferably darker, colors. Felt tip pens would work well for this exercise.
3. Outline the arteries on the diagram with the appropriate color.

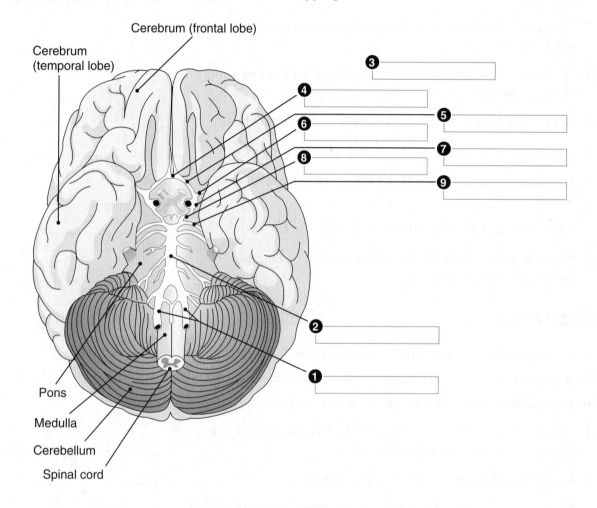

EXERCISE 14-9

Write the appropriate term in each blank from the list below.

mesenteric arch   arterial arch   cerebral arterial circle   basilar artery

anastomosis   superficial palmar arch

1. A general term describing a communication between two blood
   vessels   _____

2. An anastomosis between vessels supplying the intestines   _____

3. An anastomosis under the center of the brain formed by two
   internal carotid arteries and the basilar artery   _____

4. The vessel formed by union of the two vertebral arteries   _____

5. A vessel formed by the union of the radial and ulnar arteries   _____

6. COMPARE SUPERFICIAL AND DEEP VEINS AND GIVE EXAMPLES OF EACH TYPE.

EXERCISE 14-10

Fill in the blank after each vein—is the vein deep (D) or superficial (S)?

1. Saphenous vein _____

2. Basilic vein _____

3. Brachial vein _____

4. Femoral vein _____

5. Jugular vein _____

7. NAME THE MAIN VESSELS THAT DRAIN INTO THE SUPERIOR AND INFERIOR VENAE CAVAE.

EXERCISE 14-11: Principal Systemic Veins (Text Fig. 14-7)

Label each of the indicated veins.

1. _____

2. _____

3. _____

4. _____

5. _____

6. _____

7. _____

8. _____

9. _____

10. _____

11. _____

12. _____

13. _____

14. _____

15. _____

16. _____

17. _____

18. _____

19. _____

20. _____

21. _____

22. _____

23. _____

24. _____

25. _____

26. _____

EXERCISE 14-12: Principal Arteries and Veins of the Head (Text Figs. 14-5B and 14-7B)

Label each of the indicated arteries (bullets 1 to 11) and veins (bullets 12 to 18).

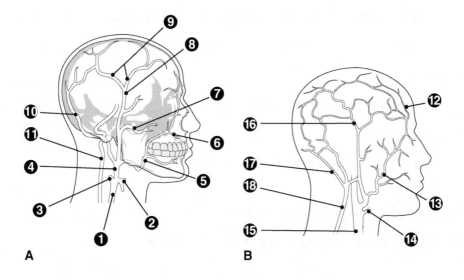

A   B

1. _____

2. _____

3. _____

4. _____

5. _____

6. _____

7. _____

8. _____

9. _____

10. _____

11. _____

12. _____

13. _____

14. _____

15. _____

16. _____

17. _____

18. _____

EXERCISE 14-13

Write the appropriate term in each blank from the list below.

cephalic vein   saphenous vein   jugular vein   gastric vein
femoral vein   lumbar vein   hepatic portal vein   common iliac vein

1. The vein that drains the area supplied by the carotid artery   _____

2. The longest vein   _____

3. A vessel that drains into the subclavian vein   _____

4. A deep vein of the thigh   _____

5. One of four pairs of veins that drain the dorsal part of the
   trunk   _____

6. A vein that sends blood to hepatic capillaries   _____

7. A vein that drains the stomach and empties into the hepatic
   portal vein   _____

8. DEFINE *VENOUS SINUS* AND GIVE SEVERAL EXAMPLES OF VENOUS SINUSES.

EXERCISE 14-14: Cranial Venous Sinuses (Text Fig. 14-7C)

1. Label each of the indicated veins and sinuses.
2. Draw arrows to indicate the direction of blood flow through the sinuses into the internal
   jugular vein (structure 9).

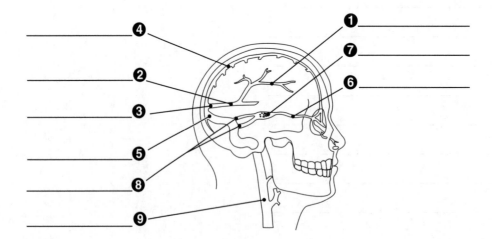

EXERCISE 14-15

Write the appropriate term in each blank from the list below.

coronary sinus   azygos vein   superior vena cava   inferior vena cava

transverse sinus   superior sagittal sinus   median cubital vein   cavernous sinus

1. A vessel that drains blood from the chest wall and empties into the superior vena cava   _____

2. The vein that receives blood draining from the head, the neck, upper extremities, and the chest   _____

3. A vein frequently used for removing blood for testing because of its location near the surface at the front of the elbow   _____

4. The large vein that drains blood from the parts of the body below the diaphragm   _____

5. The channel that drains blood from the ophthalmic vein of the eye   _____

6. The channel that drains into the confluence of sinuses   _____

7. The channel that receives blood from most of the veins of the heart wall   _____

9. DESCRIBE THE STRUCTURE AND FUNCTION OF THE HEPATIC PORTAL SYSTEM.

EXERCISE 14-16: Hepatic Portal Circulation (Text Fig. 14-8)

Label each of the indicated parts.

1. _____
2. _____
3. _____
4. _____
5. _____
6. _____
7. _____
8. _____
9. _____
10. _____
11. _____
12. _____
13. _____

10. EXPLAIN THE FORCES THAT AFFECT EXCHANGE ACROSS THE CAPILLARY WALL.

EXERCISE 14-17

Write the appropriate term in each blank from the list below.

diffusion   blood pressure   osmotic pressure

1. A force that pushes water out of the capillary _____

2. A force that moves a substance down its concentration gradient _____

3. A force that draws water into the capillary _____

11. DESCRIBE THE FACTORS THAT REGULATE BLOOD FLOW.

EXERCISE 14-18

Write the appropriate term in each blank from the list below.

vasomotor center   vasodilation   vasoconstriction   precapillary sphincter   valve

1. Structure that prevents blood from moving backward in the veins _____

2. A structure that regulates blood flow into an individual capillary _____

3. The change in a blood vessel's internal diameter caused by smooth muscle contraction _____

4. An increase in a blood vessel's internal diameter _____

5. A region of the medulla oblongata that controls contraction of the smooth muscle in blood vessel walls _____

12. DEFINE *PULSE* AND LIST THE FACTORS THAT AFFECT PULSE RATE.

EXERCISE 14-19

Fill in the blank after each of the following situations—will the pulse rate most likely increase (I) or decrease (D)?

1. A newborn baby grows older _____

2. An adult falls asleep _____

3. Thyroid gland secretion increases _____

4. A teenager runs to catch a bus _____

5. A child gets a fever _____

13. LIST THE FACTORS THAT AFFECT BLOOD PRESSURE.

EXERCISE 14-20

Fill in the blank after each of the following events—will the blood pressure most likely increase (I) or decrease (D)?

1. Decreased cardiac output _____

2. Increased blood thickness _____

3. Reduced volume of blood ejected from the heart per heartbeat _____

4. Decreased vessel elasticity (from atherosclerosis, for example) _____

5. Uncontrolled bleeding _____

6. Increased heart rate _____

7. Vasoconstriction _____

14. EXPLAIN HOW BLOOD PRESSURE IS COMMONLY MEASURED.

EXERCISE 14-21

Write the appropriate term in each blank from the list below.

viscosity   systolic pressure   diastolic pressure

sphygmomanometer   osmolarity   stethoscope

1. Term for the blood pressure reading taken after ventricular relaxation _____

2. An instrument that is used to measure blood pressure _____

3. Term for blood pressure measured after heart muscle contraction _____

4. A term that describes the thickness of a solution _____

5. The instrument used to hear changes in blood flow during the manual measurement of blood pressure _____

15. TRACE THE PATHWAY OF A BLOOD CLOT FROM THE FEMORAL VEIN TO THE PULMONARY ARTERY, REFERRING TO THE CASE STUDY.

EXERCISE 14-22

In the lines below, list all of the vessels and heart chambers that the blood clot would encounter on its journey from the femoral vein to the pulmonary artery.

_____

_____

_____

16. SHOW HOW WORD PARTS ARE USED TO BUILD WORDS RELATED TO THE BLOOD VESSELS AND CIRCULATION.

EXERCISE 14-23

Complete the following table by writing the correct word part or meaning in the space provided. Write a word that contains each word part in the Example column.

Word Part	Meaning	Example
1. _____	foot	_____
2. bar/o	_____	_____
3. _____	mouth	_____
4. hepat/o	_____	_____
5. -ectomy	_____	_____
6. _____	stomach	_____
7. _____	arm	_____
8. _____	intestine	_____
9. sphygm/o	_____	_____
10. celi/o	_____	_____

Making the Connections

The following concept map deals with the measurement and regulation of blood pressure. Each pair of terms is linked together by a connecting phrase into a sentence. The sentence should be read in the direction of the arrow. Complete the concept map by filling in the appropriate term or phrase. There is one right answer for each term. However, there are many correct answers for the connecting phrases (3 and 9).

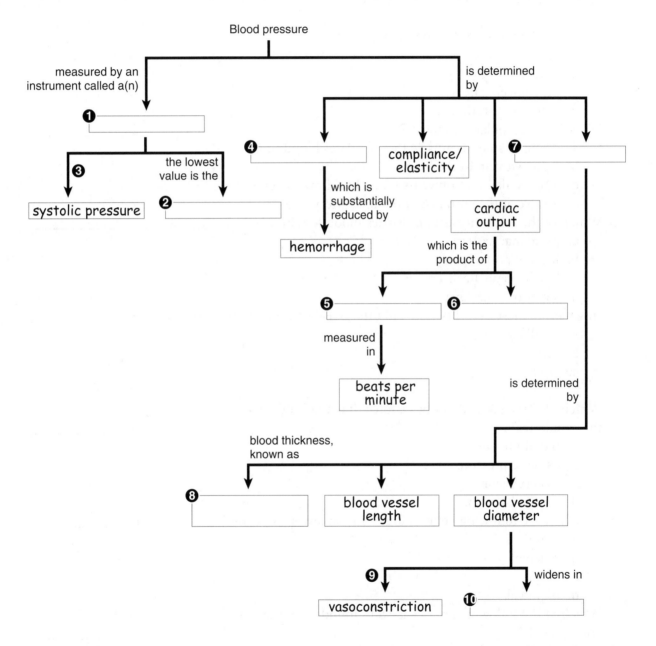

Optional Exercise: Make your own concept map/flow chart, based on the flow of blood from the left ventricle to the calf muscle. It is not necessary to include connecting statements between the terms. You can also make flow charts based on the flow of blood from the leg to the heart, or to and from the arm and/or head. Choose your own terms to incorporate into your map, or use the following list: left ventricle, femoral, anterior tibial, aortic arch, abdominal aorta, descending aorta, ascending aorta, popliteal, external iliac.

Testing Your Knowledge

BUILDING UNDERSTANDING

I. MULTIPLE CHOICE

Select the best answer and write the letter of your choice in the blank.

1. Which of the following arteries is unpaired?
    a. renal
    b. brachial
    c. brachiocephalic
    d. common carotid

    1. _____

2. What is a precapillary sphincter?
    a. a ring of smooth muscle that regulates blood flow
    b. a dilated vein in the liver
    c. a tissue flap that prevents blood backflow in veins
    d. a valve at the entrance to the iliac artery

    2. _____

3. Which of the following arteries carries blood low in oxygen?
    a. pulmonary artery
    b. hepatic portal artery
    c. brachiocephalic artery
    d. superior vena cava

    3. _____

4. In which of these vessel types would the pulse pressure be the greatest?
    a. capillary
    b. vein
    c. arteriole
    d. artery

    4. _____

5. Which of these terms describes a force drawing fluid back into the capillaries?
    a. blood pressure
    b. osmotic pressure
    c. hypertension
    d. vasoconstriction

    5. _____

6. Which of the following veins is found in the lower extremity?
    a. jugular
    b. brachial
    c. basilic
    d. popliteal

    6. _____

7. Which of the following arteries is NOT found in the cerebral arterial circle?
    a. anterior cerebral
    b. posterior communicating
    c. vertebral
    d. middle cerebral

    7. _____

8. Which of the following layers is found in arteries AND capillaries?   8. _____
   a. smooth muscle
   b. inner tunic
   c. outer tunic
   d. middle tunic

9. Which of these changes would increase blood pressure?   9. _____
   a. narrowing the blood vessels
   b. reducing the pulse rate
   c. increasing vasodilation
   d. decreasing blood viscosity

10. Which of the following is NOT a subdivision of the aorta?   10. _____
    a. thoracic aorta
    b. aortic arch
    c. pulmonary aorta
    d. abdominal aorta

11. Which two veins unite to form the inferior vena cava?   11. _____
    a. gastric veins
    b. common iliac veins
    c. jugular veins
    d. mesenteric veins

II. COMPLETION EXERCISE

Write the word or phrase that correctly completes each sentence.

1. One example of a portal system is the system that carries blood from the abdominal organs to the _____.

2. The inner, epithelial layer of blood vessels is called the _____.

3. The liver receives blood from the hepatic artery and the _____.

4. The longest vein in the body is the _____.

5. The aorta and the venae cavae are part of the group, or circuit, of blood vessels that make up the _____.

6. A large channel that drains blood low in oxygen is called a(n) _____.

7. The smallest subdivisions of arteries have thin walls in which there is little connective tissue and relatively more muscle. These vessels are _____.

8. A decrease in the diameter of a blood vessel's lumen is called _____.

9. The cerebral arterial circle is formed by a union of the internal carotid arteries and the basilar artery. Such a union of vessels is called a(n) _____.

10. The vessel that can be compressed against the lower jaw to stop bleeding in the mouth is the _____.

UNDERSTANDING CONCEPTS

I. TRUE/FALSE

For each question, write T for true or F for false in the blank to the left of each number. If a statement is false, correct it by replacing the underlined term and write the correct statement in the blanks below the question.

_____ 1. The anterior and posterior communicating arteries are part of the anastomosis supplying the brain.

_____

_____ 2. Contraction of the smooth muscle in arterioles would decrease blood pressure.

_____

_____ 3. Increased blood pressure would decrease the amount of fluid leaving the capillaries.

_____

_____ 4. The external iliac artery continues in the thigh as the femoral artery.

_____

_____ 5. The transverse sinuses receive most of the blood leaving the heart.

_____

_____ 6. Sinusoids are found in the kidney.

_____

_____ 7. Blood flow into individual capillaries is regulated by precapillary sphincters.

_____

_____ 8. Cardiac output is equal to the pulse rate x peripheral resistance.

_____

_____ 9. The inner tunic of all blood vessels is composed of muscle tissue.

_____

_____ 10. The brachiocephalic artery supplies the left arm.

_____

II. PRACTICAL APPLICATIONS

Study each discussion. Then write the appropriate word or phrase in the space provided.

➤ Group A

Ms. S, aged 68, was admitted to the hospital suffering from lightheadedness and mental confusion.

1. Physical examination showed a narrowing of a large artery on the side of the neck that carries blood to the brain. This artery is the _____.

2. Small amounts of blood could still reach Ms. S's brain through the two vertebral arteries. These join at the base of the brain to form a single artery called the

   _____.

3. Despite the impaired blood supply, blood could still access all parts of Ms. S's brain because blood could pass through the cerebral arterial circle. This connecting vessel is an example of a(n) _____.

4. Connecting vessels also link the arteries supplying the intestinal tract. These connecting vessels are collectively called the _____.

➤ Group B

1. Ms. L, aged 42, had her blood pressure examined during a routine physical. Her pressure reading was 165/100. Her diastolic pressure is thus _____.

2. The physician was very alarmed by the finding and immediately prescribed a drug to reduce the production of an enzyme produced in the kidneys that causes blood pressure to increase. This enzyme is called _____.

3. Further tests showed evidence of artery disease in several of the larger vessels. One area involved was the first portion of the aorta, called the _____.

4. The first branch off the aortic arch was also damaged. This short vessel is the

   _____.

5. The damage reflects the accumulation of fatty material in the vessel walls. The resulting roughness of the arterial wall can cause potentially fatal blood clots to form. The damaged, innermost layer of the arterial wall is known as the _____.

III. SHORT ESSAYS

1. Explain the purpose of vascular anastomoses.

   _____

   _____

   _____

2. What is the function of the hepatic portal system, and what vessels contribute to this system?

   _____

   _____

   _____

3. List the vessels a drop of blood will encounter traveling from deep within the left thigh to the right atrium.

   _____

   _____

   _____

4. Compare the structure and function of veins to that of arteries. Give at least 3 differences.

   _____

   _____

   _____

CONCEPTUAL THINKING

1. Mr. B, aged 54, is losing substantial amounts of blood due a bleeding ulcer. What will be the effect on his blood pressure? What are some physiological changes that could be made to correct this effect?

   _____

   _____

   _____

2. Ms. J has a blood pressure reading of 145/92 mm Hg. A. What is her systolic pressure? B. What is her diastolic pressure? C. Is this reading higher or lower than normal?

   _____

   _____

   _____

Expanding Your Horizons

Eat, drink, and have happy arteries. Eat more fish. Eat less fish. Drink wine. Do not drink wine. We receive conflicting messages about the effect of different foodstuffs on arterial health. The following two articles discuss some of these claims.

- Covington MB. Omega-3 fatty acids. Am Fam Physician 2004;70:133–140.
- Klatsky AL. Drink to your health? Sci Am 2003;288:74–81.

Overview

Lymph is the watery fluid that flows within the lymphatic system. It originates from the tissue fluid that is found in the minute spaces around and between the body cells. The fluid moves from the **lymphatic capillaries** through the **lymphatic vessels** and then to the **right lymphatic duct** and the **thoracic duct**. These large terminal ducts drain into the subclavian veins, adding the lymph to blood that is returning to the heart. Lymphatic capillaries resemble blood capillaries, but they begin blindly, and larger gaps between the cells make them more permeable than blood capillaries. The larger lymphatic vessels are thin walled and delicate; like some veins, they have valves that prevent backflow of lymph.

The **lymph nodes**, which are the system's filters, are composed of lymphoid tissue. These nodes remove impurities and house and process **lymphocytes**, cells active in immunity. Chief among them are the cervical nodes in the neck, the axillary nodes in the armpit, the tracheobronchial nodes near the trachea and bronchial tubes, the mesenteric nodes between the peritoneal layers, and the inguinal nodes in the groin.

In addition to the nodes, there are several organs of lymphoid tissue with somewhat different functions. For instance, the **tonsils** guard the entrance to the respiratory and digestive tracts; the **thymus** is essential for development of the immune system during early life. The **spleen** has numerous functions, including destruction of worn-out red blood cells, serving as a reservoir for blood, and producing red blood cells before birth.

Although the body is constantly exposed to pathogenic organisms, infection develops relatively rarely. This is because the body has many "lines of defense" against pathogenic invasion. Our **nonspecific (innate) defenses** are the first lines of defense, protecting us from all foreign substances. The intact **skin** and **mucous membranes** serve as mechanical barriers, as do certain **reflexes** such as sneezing and coughing. Body secretions wash away impurities and may kill bacteria as well. By the process of **inflammation**, the body tries to get rid of an irritant or to minimize its harmful effects. **Phagocytes** and **natural killer (NK) cells** act nonspecifically to destroy invaders. **Interferon** can limit viral infections. **Fever** boosts the immune system and inhibits the growth of some organisms.

The ultimate defense against disease is **specific immunity**, the means by which the body resists or overcomes the effects of a particular disease or other harmful agent. It involves reactions between foreign substances or **antigens** and the white blood cells known as **lymphocytes.** The **T cells** (T lymphocytes) produce **cell-mediated immunity.** There are different types of T cells involved in immune reactions: **cytotoxic T cells** kill infected body cells; **helper T cells** magnify all aspects of the immune response; **regulatory T cells** control the response. **Antigen-presenting cells** (dendritic cells and macrophages) participate by presenting the foreign antigen to the T cell. **B cells** (B lymphocytes), when stimulated by an antigen, multiply into **plasma cells.** These cells produce specific **antibodies**, which react with the antigen. Circulating antibodies make up the form of immunity termed **humoral immunity. Memory cells** for each lymphocyte type persist in the circulation long after the original antigen has been vanquished. These memory cells mount a rapid immune response upon subsequent antigen exposure and usually prevent infection.

Immunity may be **natural** (acquired by transfer of maternal antibodies or by contact with the disease) or **artificial** (provided by a vaccine or an immune serum). Immunity that involves production of antibodies and memory cells by the individual is termed **active immunity**; immunity acquired as a result of the transfer of antibodies to an individual from some outside source is described as **passive immunity**.

Addressing the Learning Outcomes

1. LIST THE FUNCTIONS OF THE LYMPHATIC SYSTEM.

EXERCISE 15-1

List three functions of the lymphatic system in the blanks below.

1. _____

2. _____

3. _____

EXERCISE 15-2: Lymphatic System in Relation to the Cardiovascular System (Text Fig. 15-1)

1. Label the indicated parts.
2. Color the oxygen-rich blood red, the oxygen-poor blood blue, and the lymph green.

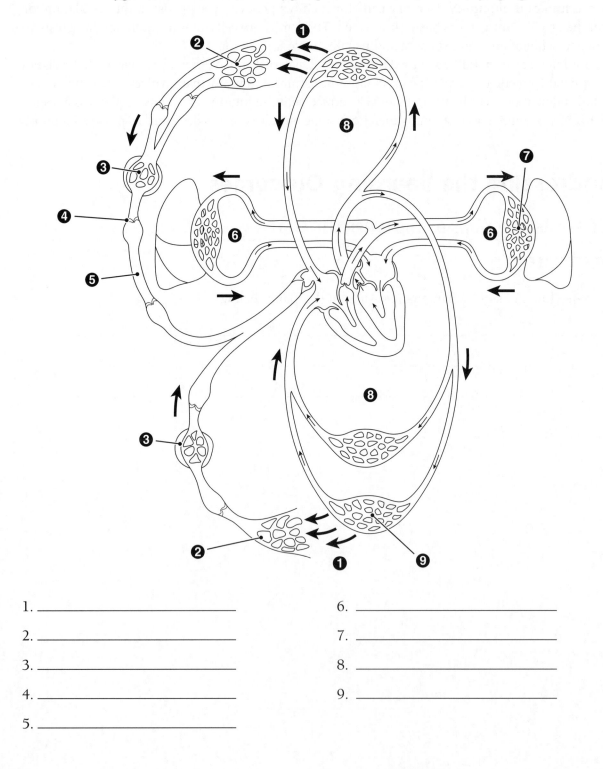

1. _____   6. _____

2. _____   7. _____

3. _____   8. _____

4. _____   9. _____

5. _____

2. EXPLAIN HOW LYMPHATIC CAPILLARIES DIFFER FROM BLOOD CAPILLARIES.

EXERCISE 15-3

Fill in the blank after each statement—does it apply to lymphatic capillaries (L), blood capillaries (B), or both (BOTH)?

1. The vessel walls are constructed of a single layer of squamous epithelial cells. _____

2. The vessel walls are very permeable, permitting the passage of large proteins. _____

3. The cells in the vessel walls are called endothelial cells. _____

4. The gap between adjacent cells in the vessel wall is very small. _____

5. Lacteals are one example of this type of vessel. _____

6. The vessels form a bridge between two larger vessels. _____

7. The capillaries drain into vessels that have valves. _____

8. The vessel transports erythrocytes. _____

3. NAME THE TWO MAIN LYMPHATIC DUCTS AND DESCRIBE THE AREA DRAINED BY EACH.

EXERCISE 15-4

Fill in the blank after each region—will the lymph drain into the right lymphatic duct (R) or the thoracic duct (T)?

1. Left hand _____

2. Right hand _____

3. Right breast _____

4. Left breast _____

5. Left leg _____

6. Right leg _____

4. LIST THE MAJOR STRUCTURES OF THE LYMPHATIC SYSTEM AND GIVE THE LOCATIONS AND FUNCTIONS OF EACH.

EXERCISE 15-5: Lymphatic System (Text Fig. 15-3)

Label the indicated parts.

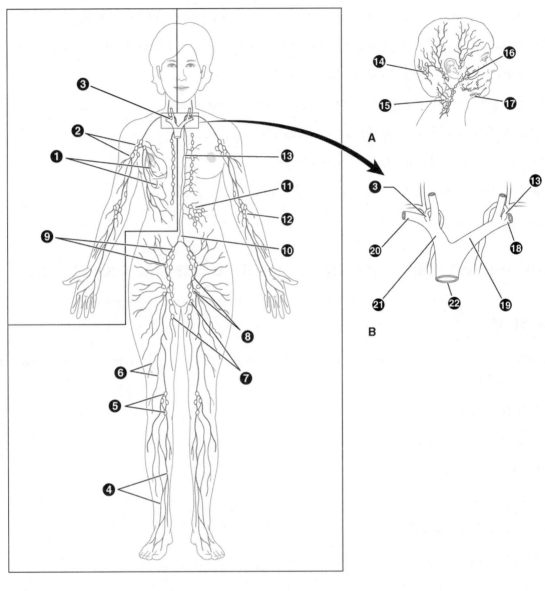

1. _____	9. _____	17. _____
2. _____	10. _____	18. _____
3. _____	11. _____	19. _____
4. _____	12. _____	20. _____
5. _____	13. _____	21. _____
6. _____	14. _____	22. _____
7. _____	15. _____	
8. _____	16. _____	

EXERCISE 15-6

Write the appropriate term in each blank from the list below.

lacteal   superficial   mesenteric nodes   cervical nodes

deep   inguinal nodes   axillary nodes

1. The nodes that filter lymph from the lower extremities and the external genitalia   _____

2. The lymph nodes located in the armpits   _____

3. Term for lymphatic vessels located near the body surface   _____

4. The lymph nodes found between the two peritoneal layers   _____

5. A specialized vessel in the small intestine wall that absorbs digested fats   _____

6. The lymph nodes located in the neck that drain certain parts of the head and neck   _____

EXERCISE 15-7

Write the appropriate term in each blank from the list below.

lymphatic capillary   right lymphatic duct   chyle   lymph

valve   subclavian vein   thoracic duct   cisterna chyli

1. The temporary storage area formed by an enlargement of the first part of the thoracic duct   _____

2. The fluid formed when tissue fluid passes from the intercellular spaces into the lymphatic vessels   _____

3. The large lymphatic vessel that drains lymph from below the diaphragm and from the left side above the diaphragm   _____

4. The milky-appearing fluid that is a combination of fat globules and lymph   _____

5. Structure that prevents backflow of fluid in lymphatic vessels   _____

6. Blind-ended, thin-walled vessel that absorbs excess tissue fluid and proteins   _____

EXERCISE 15-8: Lymph Node (Text Fig. 15-4)

Label the indicated parts.

1. _____
2. _____
3. _____
4. _____
5. _____
6. _____
7. _____
8. _____
9. _____
10. _____
11. _____
12. _____
13. _____

EXERCISE 15-9: Location of Lymphoid Tissue (Text Fig. 15-5)

1. Write the names of the different lymphoid organs on the numbered lines in different colors.
2. Color the structures on the diagram with the appropriate colors.

1. _____
2. _____
3. _____
4. _____
5. _____
6. _____
7. _____
8. _____

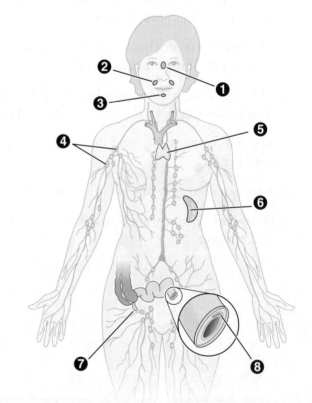

EXERCISE 15-10

Write the appropriate term in each blank from the list below.

germinal center   trabeculae   spleen   Peyer patch   MALT

palatine tonsil   lingual tonsil   pharyngeal tonsil   thymus   hilum

1. An oval lymphoid body located at the side of the soft palate   _____

2. The organ that filters blood and is located in the upper left quadrant (left hypochondriac region) of the abdomen   _____

3. A mass of lymphoid tissue at the back of the tongue   _____

4. The mass of lymphoid tissue located in the pharynx behind the nose and commonly called the adenoids   _____

5. The organ in which T cells mature   _____

6. The indented area of a lymph node where efferent lymphatic vessels exit the node   _____

7. Areas of lymphoid tissue found in mucous membranes   _____

8. An area of lymphoid tissue specifically found in the small intestine wall   _____

5. DIFFERENTIATE BETWEEN NONSPECIFIC AND SPECIFIC BODY DEFENSES AND GIVE EXAMPLES OF EACH.

EXERCISE 15-11

Write the appropriate term in each blank from the list below.

nonspecific defenses   specific defenses   natural killer cell   neutrophil

interferon   macrophage   complement

1. A substance that prevents multiplication of viruses   _____

2. A lymphocyte that nonspecifically destroys abnormal cells   _____

3. A general term describing protective responses effective against any pathogen   _____

4. A general term describing immune responses directed against an individual pathogen   _____

5. A granular leukocyte that participates in nonspecific defenses   _____

6. A set of blood proteins that carry out many different immune activities   _____

7. A phagocyte that develops from monocytes   _____

6. BRIEFLY DESCRIBE THE INFLAMMATORY REACTION.

EXERCISE 15-12

Label each of the following statements as true (T) or false (F).

1. Histamine is secreted by the damaged cells themselves. _____

2. Mast cells are similar to macrophages. _____

3. Histamine makes vessels constrict. _____

4. Leukocytes actually leave the blood vessels in order to fight infection in injured tissues. _____

5. The inflammatory exudate does not contain any cells. _____

7. DEFINE *ANTIGEN* AND *ANTIBODY*.

See Exercise 15-13, below.

8. COMPARE AND CONTRAST T CELLS AND B CELLS WITH RESPECT TO DEVELOPMENT AND TYPE OF ACTIVITY.

EXERCISE 15-13

Write the appropriate term in each blank from the list below.

foreign antigen   antibody   memory cell

plasma cell T_h cell T_{reg} cell T_c cell

1. Any external substance introduced into the body that provokes an immune response _____

2. An antibody-producing cell derived from a B cell _____

3. A cell that reduces an immune response by inhibiting or destroying activated lymphocytes _____

4. A cell that matures in the thymus and that directly destroys a foreign cell _____

5. A circulating protein also known as an immunoglobulin _____

6. A B or T cell that can rapidly activate an immune response when a previously encountered pathogen invades the body _____

7. A type of T cell that produces interleukins to stimulate immune responses _____

9. EXPLAIN THE ROLE OF ANTIGEN-PRESENTING CELLS IN SPECIFIC IMMUNITY.

EXERCISE 15-14

Write the appropriate term in each blank from the list below.

foreign antigen   MHC protein   lysosome   antibody   T cell receptor

interleukin   monocyte   neutrophil   dendritic cell

1. Macrophages are derived from this type of cell _____.

2. The organelle in macrophages that digests the foreign substance _____

3. The part of the non-self substance that is inserted into the macrophage membrane _____

4. The self-antigen inserted into the macrophage membrane _____

5. The part of the helper T cell that binds to the antigen-presenting cell _____

6. The substance released by the helper T cell after it is activated by binding to the antigen-presenting cell _____

7. A type of antigen-presenting cell with very long processes _____

10. DESCRIBE SOME PROTECTIVE EFFECTS OF AN ANTIGEN-ANTIBODY REACTION.

EXERCISE 15-15

List six ways by which the antigen–antibody reaction helps the body deal with an infection.

1. _____
2. _____
3. _____
4. _____
5. _____
6. _____

EXERCISE 15-16

Write the appropriate term in each blank from the list below.

IgG   IgM   humoral immunity   cell-mediated immunity
memory B cell   plasma cell

1. The arm of specific immunity that involves antibodies   _____

2. The arm of specific immunity that involves cytotoxic T cells   _____

3. The first type of antibody produced in an immune response   _____

4. The type of B cell that produces antibodies   _____

11. DIFFERENTIATE BETWEEN NATURAL AND ARTIFICIAL ACQUIRED IMMUNITY.

See Exercise 15-17.

12. DIFFERENTIATE BETWEEN ACTIVE AND PASSIVE IMMUNITY.

EXERCISE 15-17

For each of the following examples, state whether they involve active (ACT) or passive immunity (P), and natural (N) or artificial (ART) immunity.

1. Immunity resulting from exposure to a microbial toxin. _____ _____

2. Immunity resulting from the transfer of antibodies from mother to fetus _____
   _____

3. Immunity resulting from the HPV vaccination. _____ _____

4. Immunity resulting from the administration of antiserum. _____ _____

13. DEFINE THE TERMS *VACCINE* AND *IMMUNE SERUM*.

EXERCISE 15-18

Write the appropriate term in each blank from the list below.

toxoid   attenuation   immunization
immune serum   gamma globulin   vaccine

1. The process of reducing the virulence of a pathogen to
   prepare a vaccine   _____

2. A toxin treated with heat or chemicals to reduce its harmfulness
   so that it may be used as a vaccine   _____

3. The fraction of the blood plasma that contains antibodies   _____

4. A process designed to induce an immune response against a particular pathogen, resulting in the acquisition of artificial adaptive immunity _____

5. When this substance is administered by a medical professional, artificial passive immunity results _____

14. DESCRIBE THE SPLEEN'S FUNCTIONS AND THE CONSEQUENCES OF ITS REMOVAL, AS DESCRIBED IN THE CASE STUDY.

EXERCISE 15-19

Read Mike's case study, and review the functions of the spleen. Which of the following functions would be disrupted by Mike's splenectomy? Circle all that apply.

1. Destruction of red blood cells

2. Detection of cancer cells in lymph

3. Drainage of interstitial fluid

4. Absorption of fats from the small intestine

5. Red blood cell production in a 27-year-old

6. Response to hemorrhage

7. Detection of pathogens in blood

15. SHOW HOW WORD PARTS ARE USED TO BUILD WORDS RELATED TO THE LYMPHATIC SYSTEM.

EXERCISE 15-20

Complete the following table by writing the correct word part or meaning in the space provided. Write a word that contains each word part in the Example column.

Word Part	Meaning	Example
1. _____	gland	_____
2. lingu/o	_____	_____
3. -oid	_____	_____

Making the Connections

Map A

The following concept map deals with the structure and function of the lymphatic system. Each pair of terms is linked together by a connecting phrase. Complete the concept map by filling in the appropriate term or phrase. There is one right answer for each term. However, there are many correct answers for the connecting phrases (2, 4, 8).

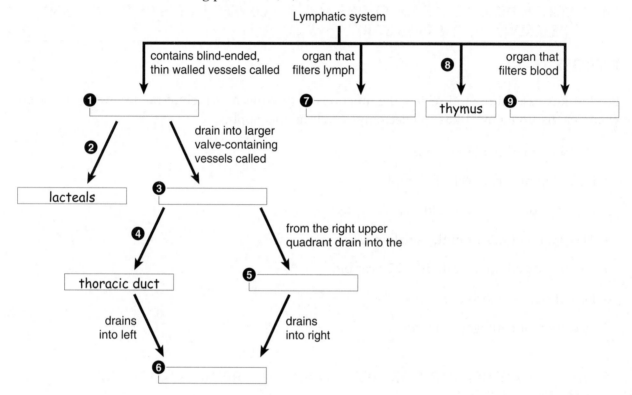

Map B

The following concept map deals with some of the processes involved in specific and nonspecific immunity. Each pair of terms is linked together by a connecting phrase into a sentence. The sentence should be read in the direction of the arrow. Complete the concept map by filling in the appropriate term or phrase. There is generally only one right answer for each term. However, there are many correct answers for the connecting phrases (4, 5, 8, 12, 15).

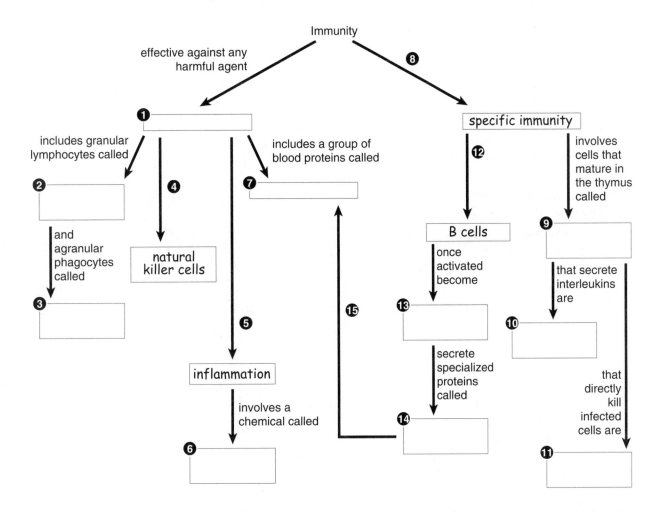

Optional Exercise: Make your own concept map/flow chart, based on the flow of lymph from a body part to the left atrium. It is not necessary to include connecting statements between the terms. For instance, you could map the flow of lymph from the right breast to the right atrium by linking the following terms: superior vena cava, right subclavian vein, right brachiocephalic vein, mammary vessels, axillary nodes, right lymphatic duct.

Testing Your Knowledge

BUILDING UNDERSTANDING

I. MULTIPLE CHOICE

Select the best answer and write the letter of your choice in the blank.

1. Which tonsil is also known as the adenoids?   1. _____
   a. palatine
   b. lingual
   c. pharyngeal
   d lymphatic
2. Which of the following is NOT a function of the spleen?   2. _____
   a. destruction of old red blood cells
   b. blood filtration
   c. blood storage
   d. chyle drainage
3. Where are the mesenteric nodes found?   3. _____
   a. in the groin region.
   b. near the trachea.
   c. between the two peritoneal layers.
   d. in the armpits.
4. Which of these organs shrinks the most in size after puberty?   4. _____
   a. cisternal chyli
   b. thymus
   c. spleen
   d. liver
5. Which of the following is a characteristic of lymphatic capillaries but
   not blood capillaries?   5. _____
   a. They contain a thin muscular layer.
   b. They are virtually impermeable to water and solutes.
   c. They are blind-ended.
   d. They do not contain any cells.
6. Which of these terms describes the enlarged portion of the thoracic duct? 6. _____
   a. cisterna chyli
   b. right lymphatic duct
   c. hilum
   d. lacteal

7. Which type of lymphocyte is involved in nonspecific immunity?   7. _____
   a. B cell
   b. natural killer cell
   c. memory T cell
   d. cytotoxic T cell

8. Which of the following describes an activity of B cells? 8. _____
   a. suppression of the immune response
   b. manufacture of antibodies
   c. direct destruction of foreign cells
   d. phagocytosis
9. Which of the following is a specific defense against infection? 9. _____
   a. skin
   b. mucus
   c. antibodies
   d. cilia
10. Which of these cells acts as an antigen-presenting cell? 10. _____
    a. macrophages
    b. cytotoxic T cells
    c. plasma cells
    d. neutrophils
11. Which of these is an action of complement proteins? 11. _____
    a. promote inflammation
    b. attract phagocytes
    c. destroy cells
    d. all of the above
12. What are interleukins? 12. _____
    a. substances in the blood that react with antigens
    b. the antibody fraction of the blood
    c. a group of nonspecific proteins needed for agglutination
    d. substances released from T_h cells that stimulate other leukocytes
13. What are MHC antigens? 13. _____
    a. bacterial proteins
    b. foreign proteins
    c. one's own proteins
    d. antibodies
14. Which of the following will result in active immunity? 14. _____
    a. immunization
    b. antiserum administration
    c. breast feeding
    d. none of the above

II. COMPLETION EXERCISE

Write the word or the phrase that correctly completes each sentence.

1. The regions within the lymph node cortex where certain lymphocytes multiply are called _____.

2. The milky-appearing lymph that drains from the small intestine is called _____.

3. The fluid that moves from tissue spaces into special collecting vessels for return to the blood is called _____.

4. Lymph from the right side of the body above the diaphragm joins the bloodstream when the right lymphatic duct empties into the _____.

5. The lymph nodes surrounding the breathing passageways may become black in individuals living in highly polluted areas. The nodes involved are the _____.

6. Nearly all of the lymph from the arm, shoulder, and breast passes through the lymph nodes known as the _____.

7. The spleen contains many cells that can engulf harmful bacteria and other foreign cells by a process called _____.

8. Circulating antibodies are responsible for the type of immunity termed _____.

9. Heat, redness, swelling, and pain are considered the classic symptoms of _____.

10. Antibodies transmitted from a mother's blood to a fetus or administered via an antiserum provide a type of short-term borrowed immunity called _____.

11. The administration of vaccine or the act of becoming infected, on the other hand, stimulates the body to produce a longer lasting type of immunity called _____.

12. The action of leukocytes in which they engulf and digest invading pathogens is known as _____.

UNDERSTANDING CONCEPTS

I. TRUE/FALSE

For each question, write T for true or F for false in the blank to the left of each number. If a statement is false, correct it by replacing the underlined term(s) and write the correct statement in the blanks below the question.

_____ 1. Lymph filtered through the mesenteric nodes will drain into the thoracic duct.

_____

_____ 2. One purpose of the lymphatic system is the absorption of protein from the small intestine.

_____

_____ 3. The spleen filters <u>lymph</u> and the lymph nodes filter <u>blood.</u>

_____

_____ 4. The <u>inguinal nodes</u> are found between the two layers of the peritoneum.

_____

_____ 5. Lacteals are a type of <u>blood capillary.</u>

_____

_____ 6. <u>Complement</u> is a substance that participates in nonspecific body defenses exclusively against viruses.

_____

_____ 7. Cytoxotic T cells participate in <u>humoral</u> immunity.

_____

_____ 8. Any immunization process involving a medical practitioner results in <u>artificial</u> immunity.

_____

_____ 9. The action of histamine in the inflammatory reaction is an example of a <u>nonspecific</u> defense.

_____

_____ 10. Immunoglobulin is another name for <u>antigens.</u>

_____

_____ 11. <u>Interferons</u> are released by helper T cells in order to stimulate the activity of other leukocytes.

_____

_____ 12. Administration of an antiserum is an example of <u>artificial, passive</u> immunity.

_____

II. PRACTICAL APPLICATIONS

Study each discussion. Then write the appropriate word or phrase in the space provided.

➤ Group A

1. Ms. L traveled in Asia for two years before starting nursing school. During the first week of classes, she noticed swelling in her right leg. She looked through her A & P textbook to try to identify the cause. She read that excess tissue fluid drains into small, blunt-ended vessels called _____.

2. To her alarm, she discovered that small worms can obstruct these vessels, causing swelling. She rushed to the hospital, where the physician palpated the small lymphoid masses found behind her knee. These masses are called the _____.

3. These masses were normal, but the lymphoid tissue masses at the top of the swollen leg were enlarged due to an infected cut in her upper thigh. These lymphoid masses are called the _____.

➤ Group B

1. Mr. R stepped on a rusty nail, resulting in a deep puncture wound. When he arrived home 2 hours later, he noticed swelling, heat, and redness in the area surrounding the painful wound. These classic signs indicate the activities of a series of defensive processes called _____.

2. Many of his signs and symptoms are due to the release of a chemical that dilates blood vessels. This chemical is called _____.

3. Mr. R went to a medical clinic for treatment. The nurse on duty asked about his immunization status. Another term for immunization is _____.

4. Mr. R had never been immunized against tetanus, so he was injected with a substance to neutralize harmful secretions produced by the tetanus bacteria. These harmful secretions are called _____.

5. The injection will produce a short-term form of immunity called _____.

III. SHORT ESSAYS

1. Trace a lymph droplet from the interstitial fluid of the lower leg to the right atrium, based on the structures shown in Figure 15-3.

_____

_____

_____

2. Discuss the role of macrophages in specific and non-specific body defenses.

_____

_____

_____

CONCEPTUAL THINKING

1. Ms. Y, a healthy 24-year old woman, is studying for her nursing finals. She has been sitting at her desk for 10 hours straight when she notices that her legs are swollen. Use your knowledge of the lymphatic system to explain the swelling, and suggest how she can prevent it in the future.

_____

_____

_____

2. Baby G was born without a thymus, but was otherwise normal. Speculate as to which aspects of her immune system will be affected by this deficiency, and which aspects will be unaffected.

_____

_____

_____

EXPANDING YOUR HORIZONS

Have you or one of your friends had the kissing disease? Infectious mononucleosis, or "mono," is an infection of lymphatic cells. It is easily transmitted between individuals living in close contact with one another (not necessarily by kissing) and is thus very common on college campuses. Learn more about this disease by reading the following articles.

- Bailey RE. Diagnosis and treatment of infectious mononucleosis. Am Fam Phys 1994;49:879–888.
- Cozad J. Infectious mononucleosis. Nurse Pract 1996;21:14–18.

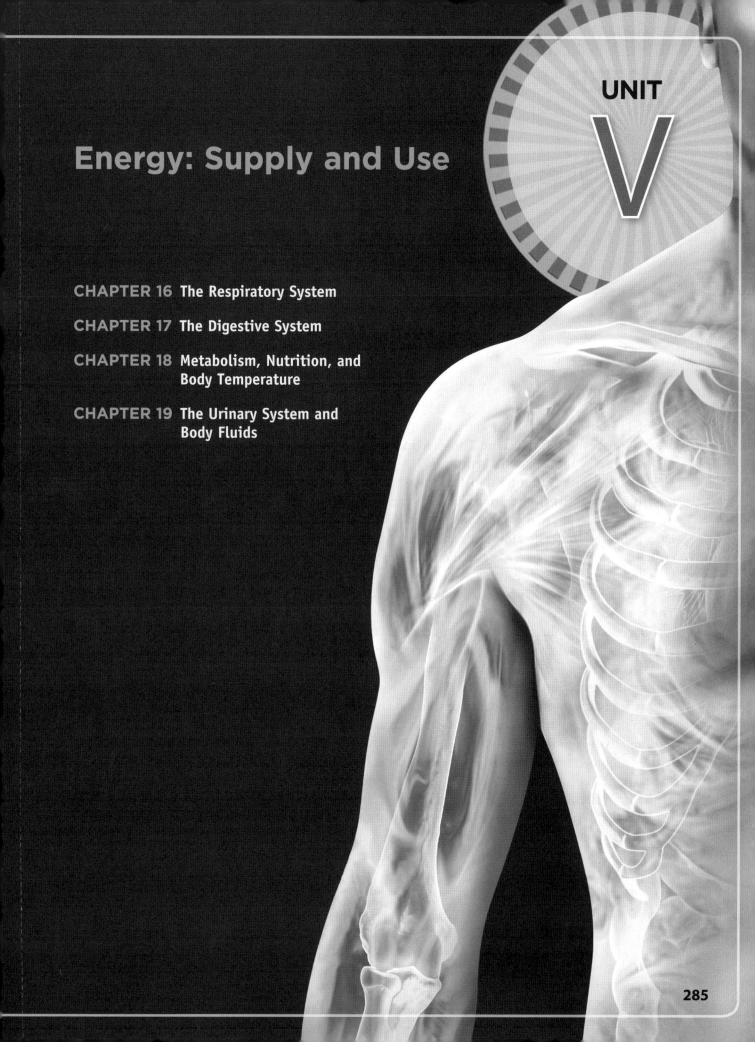

Energy: Supply and Use

UNIT

V

CHAPTER 16

The Respiratory System

Overview

Oxygen is taken into the body and carbon dioxide is released by means of the organs and passageways of the **respiratory system**. This system contains the **nasal cavities**, the **pharynx**, the **larynx**, the **trachea**, the **bronchi**, and the **lungs**.

The process of **respiration** transfers oxygen from the atmosphere to body cells and carbon dioxide from body cells to the atmosphere. It includes four stages. In terms of oxygen transfer, the first phase of respiration is **pulmonary ventilation**, which is normally accomplished by breathing. During normal, quiet breathing, air enters the lungs (**inhalation**) because the diaphragm and intercostal muscles contract to expand the thoracic cavity. Air leaves the lungs (**exhalation**) when the muscles relax. Deeper breathing requires additional muscles during both inhalation and exhalation. **External gas exchange** transfers gases between the alveoli of the lungs and the bloodstream. The specialized mechanisms of **gas transport** enable blood to carry large amounts of oxygen and carbon dioxide. Finally, **internal gas exchange** transfers gases between the blood and the tissues. Note that the latter three stages of respiration involve the cardiovascular system. The order of the stages is reversed for carbon dioxide transfer, which begins with internal gas exchange and ends with pulmonary ventilation.

Oxygen is transported to the tissues almost entirely by the **hemoglobin** in red blood cells. Some carbon dioxide is transported in the red blood cells as well, but most is converted into **bicarbonate ions** and **hydrogen ions**. Bicarbonate ions are carried in plasma, and the hydrogen ions (along with hydrogen ions from other sources) increase the acidity of the blood.

Breathing is primarily controlled by the **respiratory control centers** in the medulla and the pons of the brain stem. These centers are influenced by **chemoreceptors** located on either side of the medulla that respond to changes in the acidity of the interstitial fluid surrounding medullary neurons. The acidity reflects the concentration of carbon dioxide in arterial blood.

Addressing the Learning Outcomes

1. DEFINE RESPIRATION AND DESCRIBE THE FOUR PHASES OF RESPIRATION.

EXERCISE 16-1

Write the appropriate term in each blank from the list below.

external gas exchange   internal gas exchange   gas transport

cellular respiration   pulmonary ventilation

1. The exchange of air between the atmosphere and the alveoli   _____

2. The exchange of specific gases between the alveoli and the blood   _____

3. The exchange of specific gases between the blood and the cells   _____

4. This process involves only blood   _____

5. The process by which cells use oxygen and nutrients to generate energy   _____

2. NAME AND DESCRIBE ALL THE STRUCTURES OF THE RESPIRATORY SYSTEM.

EXERCISE 16-2: Respiratory System (Text Fig. 16-2)

Label the indicated parts.

1. _____
2. _____
3. _____
4. _____
5. _____
6. _____
7. _____
8. _____
9. _____
10. _____
11. _____
12. _____
13. _____
14. _____
15. _____
16. _____
17. _____

EXERCISE 16-3: The Larynx (Text Fig. 16-3)

1. Write the name of each labeled part on the numbered lines in different colors.
2. Color the different parts on the diagram with the corresponding color.

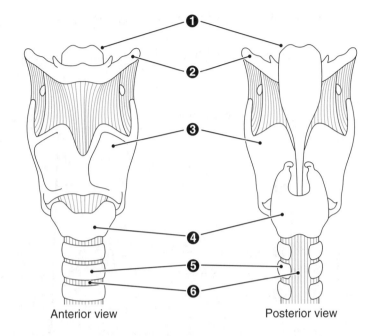

Anterior view   Posterior view

1. _____

2. _____

3. _____

4. _____

5. _____

6. _____

7. _____

8. _____

EXERCISE 16-4

Write the appropriate term in each blank from the list below.

nares   conchae   pharynx   glottis   epiglottis

larynx   parietal   bronchus   bronchiole   visceral

1. The openings of the nose   _____

2. The three projections arising from the lateral walls of each nasal cavity   _____

3. The scientific name for the voice box   _____

4. The leaf-shaped structure that helps to prevent the entrance of food into the trachea   _____

5. One of the two branches formed by division of the trachea   _____

6. The pleural layer attached to the lung   _____

7. The area below the nasal cavities that is common to both the digestive and respiratory systems   _____

8. A small air-conducting tube containing a smooth muscle layer but little or no cartilage   _____

3. EXPLAIN THE MECHANISM FOR PULMONARY VENTILATION.

EXERCISE 16-5: A Spirogram (Text Fig. 16-8)

Write the names of the different lung volumes and capacities in the boxes on the diagram.

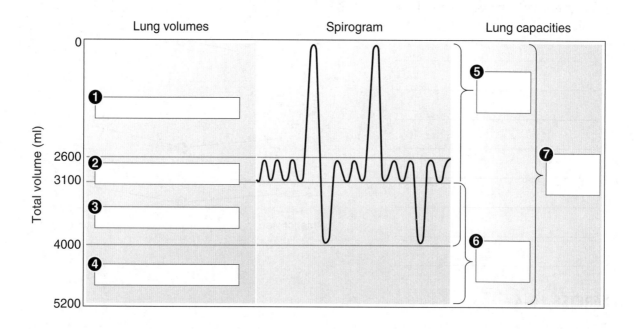

EXERCISE 16-6

Write the appropriate term in each blank from the list below.

alveoli   surfactant   inhalation   tidal volume   internal intercostals

exhalation   external intercostals   compliance   spirometer   vital capacity

1. The substance in the fluid lining the alveoli that prevents their collapse

2. The phase of pulmonary ventilation in which air is expelled from the alveoli

3. The phase of pulmonary ventilation in which the diaphragm contracts

4. Muscles involved in inhalation

5. The only respiratory structures involved in external gas exchange

6. The amount of air inhaled or exhaled during a relaxed breath

7. The ease with which the lungs and thorax can be expanded

8. The maximum volume of air that can be inhaled after maximum expiration

EXERCISE 16-7

Label each of the following statements as true (T) or false (F).

1. Inhalation is the active phase of quiet breathing   _____

2. During quiet breathing, exhalation does not require any muscle contraction   _____.

3. The diaphragm rises when it contracts.   _____

4. The external intercostal muscles contract during active exhalation   _____

5. The external intercostal muscles contract during a large inhalation   _____

6. The diaphragm relaxes during exhalation.   _____

4. DISCUSS THE PROCESSES OF INTERNAL AND EXTERNAL GAS EXCHANGE.

EXERCISE 16-8

Fill in the blanks of the following description using the following terms. Note that terms may be used more than once, and not all terms will be used.

| into | out of | body cells | diffusion |
| active transport | partial pressure gradient | osmotic gradient | alveoli |

External gas exchange transfers gases between the (1) _____ and blood. Oxygen moves (2) _____ blood and carbon dioxide moves (3) _____ blood. Internal gas exchange transfers gases between (4) _____ and blood. Oxygen moves (5) _____ blood and carbon dioxide moves (6) _____ blood. Gases move by the process of (7) _____. Each gas moves down its individual (8) _____.

5. LIST THE WAYS IN WHICH OXYGEN AND CARBON DIOXIDE ARE TRANSPORTED IN THE BLOOD.

EXERCISE 16-9

Write the appropriate term in each blank below and on the next page from the list below.

| bicarbonate ion | hemoglobin | carbonic anhydrase | carbon dioxide | 15% |
| hydrogen ion | oxygen | 10% | 75% | |

1. The gas converted into bicarbonate and hydrogen ions   _____

2. An important blood buffer produced from carbon dioxide   _____

3. The substance that carries most of the oxygen in the blood   _____

4. The gas that is more concentrated in the blood than in metabolically active tissues   _____

(continued on next page)

5. An ion that renders blood more acidic

    _____

6. The proportion of total blood carbon dioxide dissolved in plasma

    _____

7. The proportion of total blood carbon dioxide transported in the form of bicarbonate

    _____

8. The proportion of total blood carbon dioxide bound to plasma proteins and hemoglobin

    _____

6. DESCRIBE FACTORS THAT CONTROL RESPIRATION.

EXERCISE 16-10

Write the appropriate term in each blank from the list below.

hypercapnia   hydrogen ion   bicarbonate ion   phrenic nerve   vagus nerve

medulla   aortic arch   carbon dioxide   oxygen

1. The location of the main breathing regulatory center

    _____

2. A rise in the blood carbon dioxide level

    _____

3. The location of a peripheral chemoreceptor

    _____

4. The substance that acts directly on the central chemoreceptors to stimulate breathing

    _____

5. A rise in the arterial partial pressure of this gas stimulates breathing

    _____

6. The nerve that controls the diaphragm

    _____

7. DISCUSS ABNORMAL VENTILATION AND GIVE SEVERAL EXAMPLES OF ALTERED BREATHING PATTERNS.

EXERCISE 16-11

For each of the following statements, write HYPO if it refers to hypoventilation and HYPER if it refers to hyperventilation.

1. The breathing pattern that causes hypocapnia

    _____

2. The breathing pattern resulting from respiratory obstruction

    _____

3. The breathing pattern that causes hypercapnia

    _____

4. The breathing pattern that causes acidosis

    _____

5. The breathing pattern that sometimes occurs during anxiety attacks

    _____

EXERCISE 16-12

Write the appropriate term in each blank from the list below.

orthopnea   dyspnea   hyperpnea   hypoxia

hypopnea   tachypnea   apnea   hypoxemia

1. Difficult or labored breathing   _____

2. An abnormal increase in the depth and rate of breathing   _____

3. A temporary cessation of breathing   _____

4. Difficult breathing that is relieved by sitting upright   _____

5. An abnormal decrease in the depth and rate of breathing   _____

6. Rapid breathing observed during exercise   _____

7. An abnormally low oxygen partial pressure in arterial blood   _____

8. An abnormally low oxygen level in tissues   _____

8. REFERRING TO THE CASE STUDY, DISCUSS WHICH PARTS OF THE RESPIRATORY SYSTEM ARE AFFECTED BY ASTHMA.

EXERCISE 16-13

Fill in the blanks in the following discussion, referring to your textbook as needed.

In adults, the most reliable test used to diagnose asthma is (1) _____, which measures lung volumes and capacities. Emily's x-ray showed evidence of inflammation of the small airways, known as the (2) _____. Her history showed that she was sensitive to two common asthma triggers, (3) _____ and (4) _____. In order to reduce the inflammation, Emily was prescribed a low-dose (5) _____ inhaler. If this medication does not adequately control her symptoms, she will start to take an oral medication that inhibits inflammatory chemicals called (6) _____.

9. SHOW HOW WORD PARTS ARE USED TO BUILD WORDS RELATED TO RESPIRATION.

EXERCISE 16-14

Complete the following table by writing the correct word part or meaning in the space provided. Write a word that contains each word part in the Example column.

Word Part	Meaning	Example
1. _____	mouth	_____
2. spir/o	_____	_____
3. _____	larynx	_____
4. -centesis	_____	_____
5. -pnea	_____	_____
6. _____	carbon dioxide	_____
7. orth/o	_____	_____

Making the Connections

The following concept map deals with the four phases of respiration. Complete the concept map by filling in the appropriate term or phrase. There is one right answer for each term. However, there are many correct answers for the connecting phrase (5).

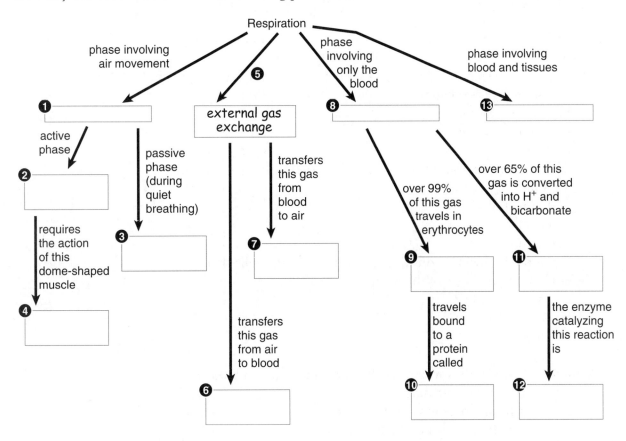

Optional Exercise: Make your own concept map/flow chart, based on the structures an oxygen molecule will pass through from the atmosphere to a tissue. Choose your own terms to incorporate into your map, or use the following list: nostrils, atmosphere, nasopharynx, oropharynx, nasal cavities, laryngeal pharynx, trachea, larynx, bronchioles, blood cell, hemoglobin, plasma, tissue, bronchi, alveoli.

Testing Your Knowledge

BUILDING UNDERSTANDING

I. MULTIPLE CHOICE

Select the best answer and write the letter of your choice in the blank.

1. During which respiratory phase does carbon dioxide diffuse out of blood? 1. _____
   a. internal gas exchange
   b. external gas exchange
   c. pulmonary ventilation
   d. none of the above

2. Which structure separates the right and left parts of the nasal cavity? 2. _____
   a. hilum
   b. bifurcation
   c. concha
   d. septum

3. Which of the following terms does NOT apply to the cells that line the conducting passages of the respiratory tract? 3. _____
   a. pseudostratified
   b. connective
   c. columnar
   d. ciliated

4. Which of these changes would result from an increase in blood carbon dioxide partial pressure? 4. _____
   a. fewer bicarbonate ions in the blood
   b. more hydrogen ions in the blood
   c. more alkaline blood
   d. hypocapnia

5. What chemical reduces surface tension in the alveoli? 5. _____
   a. surfactant
   b. bicarbonate
   c. exudate
   d. effusion

6. What is the residual volume? 6. _____
   a. The amount of air that is always in the lungs, even after a maximal expiration.
   b. The total amount of air in the lungs after a maximal inspiration.
   c. The amount of air remaining in the lungs after a normal exhalation.
   d. The amount of air that can be forced out of the lungs after a normal exhalation.

II. COMPLETION EXERCISE

Write the word or phrase that correctly completes each sentence.

1. The space between the vocal cords is called the _____.

2. An abnormal decrease in the depth and rate of respiration is termed _____.

3. A lower-than-normal partial pressure of oxygen in tissues is called _____.

4. The space between the lungs is called the _____.

5. The number of lobes in the left lung is _____.

6. The term that is used for the pressure of each gas in a mixture of gases is _____.

7. Each heme region of a hemoglobin molecule contains an inorganic element called _____.

8. The nerve that innervates the diaphragm is the _____.

UNDERSTANDING CONCEPTS

I. TRUE/FALSE

For each question, write T for true or F for false in the blank to the left of each number. If a statement is false, correct it by replacing the underlined term and write the correct statement in the blanks below the question.

_____ 1. Hypercapnia results in greater blood acidity.

_____

_____ 2. Most carbon dioxide in the blood is carried bound to hemoglobin.

_____

_____ 3. The wall of an alveolus is made of stratified squamous epithelium.

_____

_____ 4. During internal exchange of gases, oxygen moves down its concentration gradient out of blood.

_____

_____ 5. The activity of the respiratory center in the medulla can be modified by signals from a nearby brainstem region known as the midbrain.

_____

_____ 6. The alveoli become filled with exudate in patients suffering from pneumonia.

_____

_____ 7. As a result of a chronic lung disease, Ms. L's lungs do not expand very easily. Her lungs are said to be <u>more</u> compliant than normal.

_____

_____ 8. <u>Inhalation</u> during quiet breathing involves muscle contraction.

_____

_____ 9. Hyperventilation results in an <u>increase</u> of carbon dioxide in the blood.

_____

II. PRACTICAL APPLICATIONS

Study each discussion. Then write the appropriate word or phrase in the space provided.

1. Ms. L's complaints included shortness of breath, a chronic cough productive of thick mucus, and a "chest cold" of 2 months' duration. She was advised to quit smoking, because smoking irritates the tissue lining the airways. This tissue consists of a single layer of tightly packed, rectangular cells that appear to be organized into multiple layers. This type of tissue is best described as _____.

2. Symptoms in Ms. L's case were due in part to the obstruction of the air sacs by mucus. These air sacs are called _____.

3. Ms. L was told that the mucus is not moving normally out of her airways because the toxins in cigarette smoke paralyze small cell extensions that beat to create an upward current. These extensions are called _____.

4. Ms. L's respiratory function was evaluated by quantifying different lung volumes and capacities using a machine called a(n) _____.

5. Evaluation of Ms. L's respiratory function showed a reduction in the amount of air that could be moved into and out of her lungs. The amount of air that can be expelled by maximum exhalation following maximum inhalation is termed the _____.

6. The other abnormality in Ms. L's evaluation was also characteristic of her disease. There was an increase in the amount of air remaining in her lungs after a normal expiration. This amount is the _____.

III. SHORT ESSAYS

1. Are lungs passive or active players in pulmonary ventilation? Explain.

_____

_____

_____

2. Name some parts of the respiratory tract where gas exchange does NOT occur.

_____

_____

_____

CONCEPTUAL THINKING

1. a. Name the phase of respiration regulated by the respiratory control center.

_____

   b. Explain how the respiratory control center can alter this phase of respiration.

_____

_____

_____

   c. Name the chemical factor(s) that regulate(s) the activity of the respiratory control center.

_____

_____

_____

2. Use the equation below to answer the following questions.

$$CO_2 + H_2O \Leftrightarrow H_2CO_3 \Leftrightarrow H^+ + HCO_3$$

   a. Tom is holding his breath under water. What happens to the carbon dioxide content of his blood, and how does this change affect his blood acidity?

_____

   b. Notice that the arrows go in both directions, indicating the reaction can proceed in both directions. If Tom consumes a large amount of lemon juice, increasing the H^+ concentration in his blood, what do you think will happen to the amount of CO_2 in his blood? _Only consider the equation above in your answer._

_____

3. Perform the following actions as you answer the questions.
   a. Inhale as deeply as possible. Which volume do your lungs contain: the vital capacity or the total lung capacity?

   _____

   b. Beginning with a maximum inhalation, exhale all of the air you can. Which volume did you exhale: the vital capacity or the total lung capacity?

   _____

   c. Breathe quietly for a few minutes, and stop after a normal exhale. Which volume remains in your lungs: the functional residual capacity or the residual volume?

   _____

   d. Breathe quietly for a few minutes, and then actively exhale all of the air you can. Which volume remains in your lungs: the functional residual capacity or the residual volume?

   _____

Expanding Your Horizons

Everyone would agree that oxygen is a very useful molecule. Commercial enterprises, working on the premise that More is Better, market water supplemented with extra oxygen. They claim that consumption of hyperoxygenated water increases alertness and exercise performance. Do these claims make sense? Do we obtain oxygen from the lungs or from the digestive tract? A logical extension of this premise is that soda pop, supplemented with carbon dioxide, would increase carbon dioxide in the blood and thus increase the breathing rate. Is this true? You can read about another oxygen gimmick, oxygen bars, on the Web site of the Food and Drug Administration.

- Bren L. Oxygen bars: is a breath of fresh air worth it? 2002. Available at: http://permanent.access.gpo.gov/lps1609/www.fda.gov/fdac/features/2002/602_air.html

CHAPTER 17

The Digestive System

Overview

The food we eat is made available to cells throughout the body by the complex processes of **digestion** and **absorption**. These are the functions of the **digestive system**, composed of the **digestive tract** and the **accessory organs**.

The digestive tract, consisting of the **mouth**, the **pharynx**, the **esophagus**, the **stomach**, and the small and large **intestines**, forms a continuous passageway in which ingested food is prepared for use by the body and waste products are collected to be expelled from the body. The accessory organs, the **salivary glands**, **liver**, **gallbladder**, and **pancreas**, manufacture and store various enzymes and other substances needed in digestion.

Digestion begins in the mouth with the digestion of starch. It continues in the stomach, where protein digestion begins, and is completed in the small intestine. Most absorption of digested food also occurs in the small intestine through small projections of the lining called **villi**. The products of carbohydrate (monosaccharides) and protein (amino acids) digestion are absorbed into capillaries, but most products of fat digestion (glycerol and most fatty acids) are absorbed into **lacteals**. The process of digestion is controlled by both nervous and hormonal mechanisms, which regulate the secretory activity of the digestive organs and the rate at which food moves through the digestive tract.

Addressing the Learning Outcomes

1. NAME THE THREE MAIN FUNCTIONS OF THE DIGESTIVE SYSTEM.

EXERCISE 17-1

List the three main functions of the digestive system in the blanks below in the order in which they occur.

1. _____

2. _____

3. _____

2. DESCRIBE THE FOUR LAYERS OF THE DIGESTIVE TRACT WALL.

EXERCISE 17-2: The Digestive Tract Wall (Text Fig. 17-1)

1. Write the names of the four layers of the digestive tract wall in boxes 1 to 4 on the diagram, using four light colors. Lightly shade each layer with the appropriate color on the diagram.
2. Write the names of the structures in the appropriate lines.

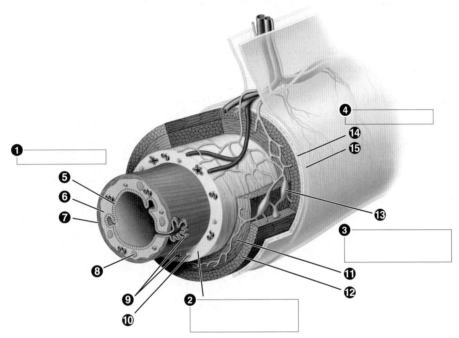

1. _____
2. _____
3. _____
4. _____
5. _____
6. _____
7. _____
8. _____
9. _____
10. _____
11. _____
12. _____
13. _____
14. _____
15. _____

EXERCISE 17-3

Write the appropriate term in each blank from the list below.

mucosa   muscularis externa   submucosa

serosa   squamous epithelium   simple columnar epithelium

1. The digestive tract layer in contact with the intestinal contents   _____

2. The visceral peritoneum attached to the surface of a digestive organ   _____

3. The layer of connective tissue beneath the mucous membrane in the wall of the digestive tract   _____

4. The layer of the digestive tract wall that is responsible for peristalsis   _____

5. The type of epithelial tissue lining the esophagus   _____

6. The type of epithelial tissue lining the stomach   _____

3. NAME AND LOCATE THE TWO MAIN LAYERS AND THE SUBDIVISIONS OF THE PERITONEUM.

EXERCISE 17-4: Abdominopelvic Cavity and Peritoneum (Text Fig. 17-2)

1. Write the names of the abdominal organs on the appropriate numbered lines 1 to 9 in different colors. Use the same color for parts 3 and 4.
2. Color the organs on the diagram with the appropriate colors.
3. Label the parts of the peritoneum (lines 10 to 15). Color the greater and lesser peritoneal cavities in contrasting colors.

1. _____
2. _____
3. _____
4. _____
5. _____
6. _____
7. _____
8. _____
9. _____
10. _____
11. _____
12. _____
13. _____
14. _____
15. _____

☐ Greater peritoneal cavity
☐ Lesser peritoneal cavity

EXERCISE 17-5

Write the appropriate term in each blank from the list below.

parietal peritoneum   visceral peritoneum   greater peritoneal cavity

mesocolon   greater omentum   lesser omentum   lesser peritoneal cavity

1. The innermost layer of the serous membrane in contact with abdominal organs

   _____

2. The outer layer of the serous membrane lining the abdominopelvic cavity

   _____

3. The subdivision of the peritoneum that contains fat and hangs over the front of the intestines

   _____

4. The subdivision of the peritoneum extending between the stomach and liver

   _____

5. The subdivision of the peritoneum that extends from the colon to the posterior abdominal wall

   _____

6. The fluid-filled cavity that extends behind the stomach to the liver and the posterior portion of the diaphragm

   _____

4. NAME AND LOCATE THE DIFFERENT TYPES OF TEETH.

EXERCISE 17-6: The Mouth (Text Fig. 17-4).

1. Write the names of the teeth on the appropriate lines 1 to 6 in different colors. Use the same color to label parts 5 and 6.
2. Color all of the teeth with the appropriate colors.
3. Label the other parts of the mouth.

1. _____

2. _____

3. _____

4. _____

5. _____

6. _____

7. _____

8. _____

9. _____

10. _____

11. _____

12. _____

13. _____

14. _____

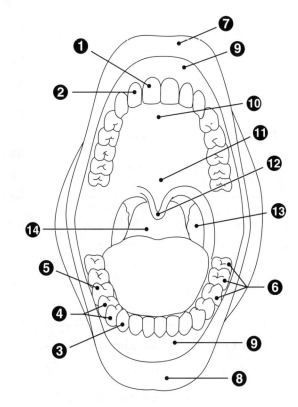

EXERCISE 17-7: A Molar Tooth (Text Fig. 17-5)

1. Write the names of the two divisions of a tooth in the numbered boxes.
2. Write the names of the parts of the tooth and gums on the appropriate numbered lines in different colors. Use the same color for parts 3 and 4, for 6 and 7, and for 8 and 9. Use a dark color for structure 8, because it will be outlined.

3. _____

4. _____

5. _____

6. _____

7. _____

8. _____

9. _____

10. _____

EXERCISE 17-8

Write the appropriate term in each blank from the list below.

| deglutition | mastication | incisors | enamel | periodontal ligament |
| deciduous | cuspids | dentin | gingiva | cementum |

1. Term that describes the baby teeth, based on the fact that they are lost

   _____

2. The process of chewing

   _____

3. The act of swallowing

   _____

4. The medical term for the gum

   _____

5. The eight cutting teeth located in the front part of the oral cavity

   _____

6. A calcified substance making up most of the tooth structure

   _____

7. The fibrous connective tissue joining the tooth to the tooth socket

   _____

8. The calcified substance coating the tooth

   _____

5. NAME AND DESCRIBE THE FUNCTIONS OF THE DIGESTIVE TRACT ORGANS.

EXERCISE 17-9: Digestive System (Text Fig. 17-3)

1. Trace the path of food through the digestive tract by labeling parts 1 to 12. You can color all of these structures orange.
2. Write the names of the accessory organs and ducts on the appropriate lines in different colors. You may also have to refer to Figure 17-8 in your textbook.
3. Color the accessory organs on the diagram with the appropriate colors.

1. _____
2. _____
3. _____
4. _____
5. _____
6. _____
7. _____
8. _____
9. _____
10. _____
11. _____
12. _____
13. _____
14. _____
15. _____
16. _____
17. _____
18. _____
19. _____

EXERCISE 17-10: Longitudinal Section of the Stomach (Text Fig. 17-6)

1. Label the parts of the stomach, esophagus, and duodenum (parts 1 to 7).
2. Label the layers of the stomach wall (parts 8 to 11). You can use colors to highlight the different muscular layers.
3. Label the two stomach curvatures (labels 12 and 13).

1. _____
2. _____
3. _____
4. _____
5. _____
6. _____
7. _____
8. _____
9. _____
10. _____
11. _____
12. _____
13. _____

EXERCISE 17-11: The Intestines (Text Fig. 17-7A)

Label the indicated parts.

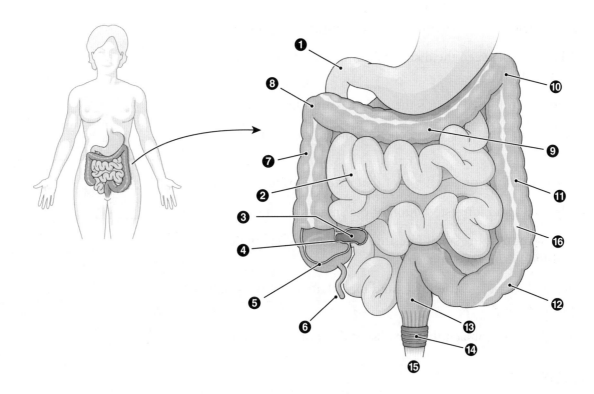

1. _____

2. _____

3. _____

4. _____

5. _____

6. _____

7. _____

8. _____

9. _____

10. _____

11. _____

12. _____

13. _____

14. _____

15. _____

16. _____

EXERCISE 17-12

Write the appropriate term in each blank from the list below.

ileum　hard palate　soft palate　epiglottis　pyloric sphincter

LES　rugae　chyme　duodenum　jejunum

1. The valve between the distal end of the stomach and the small intestine _____

2. The structure that guards the entrance into the stomach _____

3. A structure that covers the opening of the larynx during swallowing _____

4. The part of the oral cavity roof that extends to form the uvula _____

5. The final, and longest, section of the small intestine _____

6. The section of the small intestine that receives gastric juices and food from the stomach _____

7. The mixture of gastric juices and food that enters the small intestine _____

8. Folds in the stomach that are absent if the stomach is full _____

EXERCISE 17-13

Write the appropriate term in each blank from the list below.

villi　teniae coli　cecum　transverse colon

vermiform appendix　lacteal　rectum　ileocecal valve

1. The part of the large intestine just proximal to the anus _____

2. The small blind tube attached to the first part of the large intestine _____

3. The sphincter that prevents food moving from the large intestine into the small intestine _____

4. Fingerlike extensions of the mucosa in the small intestine _____

5. A blind-ended lymphatic vessel that absorbs fat _____

6. Bands of longitudinal muscle in the large intestine _____

7. The portion of the large intestine that extends across the abdomen _____

8. The most proximal part of the large intestine _____

6. NAME AND DESCRIBE THE FUNCTIONS OF THE ACCESSORY ORGANS OF DIGESTION.

EXERCISE 17-14: Accessory Organs of Digestion (Text Fig. 17-9)

1. Write the names of the labeled parts on the appropriate lines in different colors.
2. Color the structures on the diagram.

1. _____
2. _____
3. _____
4. _____
5. _____
6. _____
7. _____
8. _____
9. _____
10. _____

EXERCISE 17-15

Write the appropriate term in each blank from the list below.

parotid glands   submandibular glands   sublingual glands   gallbladder

liver   pancreas

1. The gland that secretes bicarbonate and digestive enzymes _____

2. An organ that stores nutrients and releases them as needed into the bloodstream _____

3. The accessory organ that stores bile _____

4. The salivary glands that are inferior and anterior to the ear _____

5. Glands found just under the tongue that secrete into the oral cavity _____

7. DESCRIBE HOW BILE TRAVELS INTO THE DIGESTIVE TRACT AND FUNCTIONS IN DIGESTION.

EXERCISE 17-16

Write the appropriate term in each blank from the list below.

common bile duct   urea   cystic duct   pancreatic duct   bile

bicarbonate   bilirubin   glycogen   common hepatic duct

1. A substance that emulsifies fat
   _____

2. The form in which glucose is stored in the liver
   _____

3. A waste product produced from the destruction of red blood cells
   _____

4. A waste product synthesized by the liver as a result of protein metabolism
   _____

5. The duct connecting the hepatic duct to the gallbladder
   _____

6. The duct that connects to the pancreatic duct
   _____

7. The duct that carries bile from both lobes of the liver to the common bile duct
   _____

8. EXPLAIN THE ROLE OF ENZYMES IN DIGESTION AND GIVE EXAMPLES OF THESE ENZYMES.

EXERCISE 17-17

Write the appropriate term in each blank from the list below.

protein   hydrolysis   fat   nuclease   pepsin

sodium bicarbonate   lipase   maltose   trypsin   maltase

1. An enzyme that acts on a particular type of disaccharide
   _____

2. A substance (NOT an enzyme) released into the small intestine that neutralizes the acidity in chime
   _____

3. A substance that digests DNA
   _____

4. A pancreatic enzyme that splits proteins into amino acids
   _____

5. An enzyme secreted into the stomach that splits proteins into amino acids
   _____

6. The splitting of food molecules by the addition of water
   _____

7. Lipase participates in the digestion of this nutrient
   _____

8. The nutrient type that is partially digested by gastric juice
   _____

9. NAME THE DIGESTION PRODUCTS OF FATS, PROTEINS, AND CARBOHYDRATES.

EXERCISE 17-18

Fill in the blank after each statement—does it apply to carbohydrates (C), proteins (P), or fats (F)?

1. This nutrient type is digested into sugars. _____

2. This nutrient type is digested into amino acids. _____

3. This nutrient type is digested into glycerol and fatty acids. _____

4. This nutrient type is partially digested in the stomach in both children and adults.
_____

5. This nutrient type can be broken down into disaccharides. _____

10. DEFINE *ABSORPTION* AND STATE HOW VILLI FUNCTION IN ABSORPTION.

EXERCISE 17-19

Write a definition of *absorption* in the space below.

_____

EXERCISE 17-20

Label each of the following statements as true (T) or false (F).

1. Digested carbohydrates are absorbed into lacteals. _____

2. Villi are small extensions the plasma membranes of individual intestinal cells. _____

3. Villi are folds in the mucosa, each composed of many cells. _____

4. Most digested fats are absorbed into lacteals. _____

11. EXPLAIN THE USE OF FEEDBACK IN REGULATING DIGESTION AND GIVE SEVERAL EXAMPLES.

EXERCISE 17-21

Complete the following discussion by choosing one of the terms in brackets after each blank.

Digestion is regulated by (1) _____ (negative, positive) feedback, a type of feedback that maintains homeostasis. For instance, (2) _____ (gastrin, secretin) is released from duodenal cells in response to (3) _____ (increased, decreased) acidity in the intestine. This hormone, in turn, stimulates (4) _____ (bile, bicarbonate) release from the pancreas, which neutralizes the change in acidity. Once the intestinal pH returns to normal, the release of this hormone is (5) _____ (increased, decreased).

12. LIST SEVERAL HORMONES INVOLVED IN REGULATING DIGESTION.

EXERCISE 17-22

Write the appropriate term in each blank from the list below.

leptin   gastrin   gastric-inhibitory peptide

cholecystokinin (CCK)   secretin

1. A hormone released from fat cells that inhibits appetite   _____

2. A duodenal hormone that stimulates insulin release   _____

3. A hormone that stimulates the secretion of gastric juice and increases stomach motility   _____

4. An intestinal hormone that causes the gallbladder to contract, releasing bile   _____

5. A duodenal hormone that controls bicarbonate production in the pancreas   _____

13. USING THE CASE STUDY, DESCRIBE THE COLONOSCOPY PROCEDURE AND ITS ROLE IN DIAGNOSING CERTAIN COLON DISORDERS.

EXERCISE 17-23

Label each of the following statements as true (T) or false (F).

a. You should only get a colonoscopy if you have family members with colon cancer.   _____

b. Traditional colonoscopy uses an endoscope.   _____

c. Virtual colonoscopies use a small camera inside a pill that the patient swallows.   _____

d. All individuals over 50 years of age should consider getting a colonoscopy.   _____

14. SHOW HOW WORD PARTS ARE USED TO BUILD WORDS RELATED TO DIGESTION.

EXERCISE 17-24

Complete the following table by writing the correct word part or meaning in the space provided. Write a word that contains each word part in the Example column.

Word Part	Meaning	Example
1. _____	starch	_____
2. mes/o-	_____	_____
3. _____	intestine	_____
4. chole	_____	_____
5. bil/i	_____	_____
6. _____	bladder, sac	_____
7. _____	stomach	_____
8. _____	away from	_____
9. hepat/o	_____	_____
10. lingu/o	_____	_____

Making the Connections

The following concept map deals with the structure and regulation of the gastrointestinal system. Each pair of terms is linked together by a connecting phrase into a sentence. Complete the concept map by filling in the appropriate term or phrase. There is one right answer for each term (1, 2, 4, 7, 8, 12, 13). However, there are many correct answers for the connecting phrases. Write the connecting phrases along the arrows if possible. If your phrases are too long, you may want to write them in the margins or on a separate sheet of paper. Can you think of any other phrases to connect the terms? For instance, how could you connect "CCK" with "pancreas"?

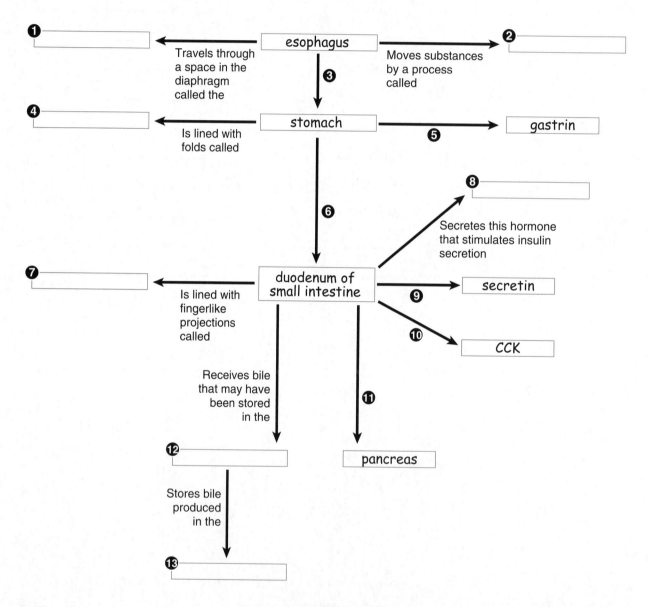

Optional Exercise: Make your own concept map, based on the three processes of digestion and how they apply to proteins, sugars, and fats. Choose your own terms to incorporate into your map, or use the following list: digestion, absorption, elimination, stomach, small intestine, large intestine, fats, carbohydrates, proteins, amylase, lipase, bile, hydrochloric acid, pepsin, trypsin, peptidase, maltase.

Testing Your Knowledge

BUILDING UNDERSTANDING

I. MULTIPLE CHOICE

Select the best answer and write the letter of your choice in the blank.

1. Which teeth would NOT be found in a 20-year-old male?
   a. bicuspid
   b. cuspid
   c. deciduous
   d. incisor

1. _____

2. Which of the following is the correct order of tissue from the innermost to the outermost layer in the wall of the digestive tract?
   a. submucosa, serous membrane, smooth muscle, mucous membrane
   b. smooth muscle, serous membrane, mucous membrane, submucosa
   c. serous membrane, smooth muscle, submucosa, mucosa
   d. mucous membrane, submucosa, smooth muscle, serous membrane

2. _____

3. Where is the parotid gland located?
   a. inferior and anterior to the ear
   b. under the tongue
   c. in the cheek
   d. in the oropharynx

3. _____

4. Which of the following is NOT a portion of the peritoneum?
   a. mesocolon
   b. mesentery
   c. hiatus
   d. greater omentum

4. _____

5. What are the two active chemicals found in gastric juice?
   a. amylase and pepsin
   b. pepsin and hydrochloric acid
   c. maltase and secretin
   d. bile and trypsin

5. _____

6. Which of these chemicals is released in response to gastric-inhibitory peptide?
   a. pepsin
   b. insulin
   c. bicarbonate
   d. gastrin

6. _____

7. Where does most fat digestion occur in adults?
   a. mouth
   b. stomach
   c. small intestine
   d. transverse colon

7. _____

8. Which of the following does NOT occur in the mouth?　　8. _____
   a. mastication
   b. digestion of starch
   c. absorption of nutrients
   d. ingestion
9. Which of the following is an enzyme?　　9. _____
   a. bile
   b. gastrin
   c. trypsin
   d. secretin
10. Which of the following is associated with the intestine?　　10. _____
   a. rugae
   b. lacteals
   c. LES
   d. greater curvature

II. COMPLETION EXERCISE

Write the word or phrase that correctly completes each sentence.

1. The process by which ingested nutrients are broken down into smaller components is called _____.

2. The lower part of the colon bends into an S shape, so this part is called the _____.

3. A temporary storage section for indigestible and unabsorbable waste products of digestion is the _____.

4. The wavelike movement created by alternating muscle contractions is called _____.

5. The large intestine can be examined using a type of endoscope called a(n) _____.

6. Most digestive juices contain substances that cause the chemical breakdown of foods without entering into the reaction themselves. These catalytic agents are _____.

7. The portion of the peritoneum extending between the stomach and liver is called the _____.

8. The process of swallowing is called _____.

9. Teeth are largely composed of a calcified substance called _____.

10. The esophagus passes through the diaphragm at a point called the _____.

11. The hormone that stimulates gallbladder contraction is called _____.

12. Small projecting folds in the plasma membrane of intestinal epithelial cells are called _____.

13. The stomach enzyme involved in protein digestion is called _____.

UNDERSTANDING CONCEPTS

I. TRUE/FALSE

For each question, write T for true or F for false in the blank to the left of each number. If a statement is false, correct it by replacing the underlined term and write the correct statement in the blanks below the question.

_____ 1. There are <u>32</u> deciduous teeth.

_____

_____ 2. The layer of the peritoneum attached to the liver is part of the <u>visceral</u> peritoneum.

_____

_____ 3. The LES restricts the passage of stomach contents into the <u>duodenum</u>.

_____

_____ 4. Ms. Q is deficient in lactase. She will be unable to digest some <u>carbohydrates</u>.

_____

_____ 5. Trypsin is secreted by the <u>gastric glands</u>.

_____

_____ 6. Increased acidity in the chyme could be neutralized by the actions of the hormone <u>gastrin</u>.

_____

_____ 7. Fats are absorbed into <u>blood capillaries</u> in the intestinal villi.

_____

_____ 8. The middle section of the small intestine is called the <u>jejunum</u>.

_____

_____ 9. Folds in the stomach wall are called <u>villi</u>.

_____

_____ 10. The <u>common bile</u> duct delivers bile from the liver and gallbladder into the duodenum.

_____

_____ 11. Amylase is involved in the digestion of <u>carbohydrates</u>.

_____

_____ 12. The <u>pancreas</u> is responsible for the synthesis of urea.

_____

II. PRACTICAL APPLICATIONS

Study each discussion. Then write the appropriate word or phrase in the space provided.

1. Mr. P, age 42, came to the clinic complaining of pain in the "pit of his stomach." He was a tense man who divided up his long working hours with coffee and cigarette breaks. When asked about his alcohol consumption, Mr. C mentioned that he drank 3 or 4 beers and a glass of wine each night, and significantly more on the weekends. Endoscopy showed inflammation of the innermost layer of the stomach. This layer is called the _____.

2. A damaged area was also found in the most proximal part of the small intestine. This section of the small intestine is called the _____.

3. Mr. P was diagnosed with an ulcer and given a prescription for antibiotics. The antibiotics will treat the bacterium involved in ulcer formation. These bacteria are named after the most distal portion of the stomach, the _____.

4. A second medication inhibits a hormone that stimulates gastric gland activity. This hormone is called _____.

5. The physician had almost completed her physical exam of Mr. P when she felt the edge of his liver about 5 cm (2 in) below the ribs. She also noticed that the whites of his eyes were tinged with yellow. The yellowish coloration results from the buildup of a yellowish pigment in blood. This pigment results from the breakdown of red blood cells and is known as _____.

6. Based on her clinical findings and Mr. P's self-reported alcohol abuse, the physician suspected that Mr. P has cirrhosis, a chronic liver disease. Further testing also revealed a partial blockage of the duct leading from the gall bladder. This duct is the _____.

III. SHORT ESSAYS

1. Describe some features of the small intestine that increase the surface area for absorption of nutrients.

   _____

   _____

   _____

   _____

2. List four differences between the digestion and/or absorption of fats and proteins.

   _____

   _____

   _____

   _____

CONCEPTUAL THINKING

1. Ms. M is taking a drug that blocks the action of cholecystokinin. Discuss the impact of this drug on digestion.

_____

_____

_____

_____

2. Is bile an enzyme? Explain your answer.

_____

_____

_____

_____

Expanding Your Horizons

Both inflammatory bowel disease and Crohn disease are autoimmune disorders of the gastrointestinal tract that frequently develop in young adults. The most common treatments attempt to reduce the inflammatory response, but they have significant side effects, including significant weight gain and fatigue. Dr. Joel Weinstock has developed an alternative treatment—drinking worm cocktails. The hypothesis is that the worms secrete substances that inhibit the immune response. Everyone wins because the immune system leaves both the worms and the intestinal lining alone. You can read more about this work on Dr. Weinstock's Web site, or in the article listed below.

- The Joel Weinstock Lab. Available at:
  http://sackler.tufts.edu/Academics/Degree-Programs/PhD-Programs/Faculty-Research-Pages/Joel-Weinstock.aspx
- Weinstock JV, Elliott DE. Helminths and the IBD hygiene hypothesis. Inflamm Bowel Dis 2009(January);15:128–133. Available at: http://onlinelibrary.wiley.com/doi/10.1002/ibd.20633/full

CHAPTER 18

Metabolism, Nutrition, and Body Temperature

Overview

The nutrients that reach the cells following digestion and absorption are used to maintain life. All the chemical reactions that occur within the cells make up **metabolism**, which includes **catabolism**, reactions that break down large molecules into smaller ones, and **anabolism**, reactions that build large molecules from smaller ones. Some catabolic reactions are specialized to produce energy in the form of ATP. The catabolism of glucose requires two major stages. The first stage, **glycolysis**, is described as **anaerobic** (does not require oxygen) and produces a small amount of energy. The end product of glycolysis is called **pyruvic acid**. Pyruvic acid, fatty acids, or even amino acids can be completely broken down by mitochondria to yield large amounts of ATP. These reactions are **aerobic** (requiring oxygen) and can be described as nutrient oxidation or **cellular respiration**.

By the various metabolic pathways, the breakdown products of food can be built into substances needed by the body. The **essential** amino acids and fatty acids cannot be manufactured internally and must be ingested in food. **Minerals** and **vitamins** are also needed in the diet for health. A balanced diet includes carbohydrates, proteins, and fats consumed in amounts relative to individual activity levels.

The rate at which energy is released from nutrients is termed the **metabolic rate**. It is affected by many factors including age, size, sex, activity, and hormones. Some of the energy in nutrients is released as heat. Heat production is greatly increased during periods of increased muscular or glandular activity. Most heat is lost through the skin, but heat is also dissipated through exhaled air and eliminated waste products (urine and feces). The **hypothalamus** maintains body temperature at approximately 37°C (98.6°F) by altering blood flow through the surface blood vessels and the activity of sweat glands and muscles.

Addressing the Learning Outcomes

1. DIFFERENTIATE BETWEEN CATABOLISM AND ANABOLISM.

EXERCISE 18-1

Fill in the blank after each statement—does it apply to catabolism (C) or to anabolism (A)?

1. The metabolic breakdown of complex compounds _____

2. The metabolic building of simple compounds into substances
   needed by cells _____

3. This process usually releases energy _____

2. DIFFERENTIATE BETWEEN THE ANAEROBIC AND AEROBIC PHASES OF GLUCOSE CATABOLISM AND GIVE THE END PRODUCTS AND THE RELATIVE AMOUNT OF ENERGY RELEASED BY EACH.

EXERCISE 18-2

Fill in the blank after each statement—does it apply to the anaerobic phase (AN) or to the aerobic phase (AE) of glucose catabolism?

1. This process generates 2 ATP per glucose molecule _____

2. This process generates about 30 ATP per glucose molecule _____

3. The end products are carbon dioxide and water _____

4. The end product is pyruvic acid _____

5. This process can occur in the absence of oxygen _____

6. This process requires oxygen _____

7. This process occurs first _____

3. DEFINE *METABOLIC RATE* AND NAME SEVERAL FACTORS THAT AFFECT THE METABOLIC RATE.

EXERCISE 18-3

Write a definition for each term in the blanks provided.

1. Metabolism _____

_____

2. Metabolic rate _____

_____

3. Basal metabolism _____

_____

4. EXPLAIN HOW CARBOHYDRATES, FATS, AND PROTEINS ARE METABOLIZED FOR ENERGY.

See Exercise 18-4.

5. COMPARE THE ENERGY CONTENTS OF FATS, PROTEINS, AND CARBOHYDRATES.

EXERCISE 18-4

Write the appropriate term in each blank from the list below.

glycolysis	pyruvic acid	glycerol	lactic acid
glycogen	deamination	fat	protein

1. The storage form of glucose _____

2. A modification of amino acids that occurs before they can be oxidized for energy _____

3. An intermediate product of glucose catabolism that can be completely oxidized within the mitochondria _____

4. An organic substance produced from pyruvic acid during intense exercise _____

5. The nutrient type that generates the most energy per gram _____

6. A product of fat digestion that can be used for energy _____

7. The nutrient type that does not have a specialized storage form _____

6. DEFINE *ESSENTIAL AMINO ACID.*

See Exercise 18-5.

7. EXPLAIN THE ROLES OF MINERALS AND VITAMINS IN NUTRITION AND GIVE EXAMPLES OF EACH.

EXERCISE 18-5

Write the appropriate term in each blank from the list below.

essential amino acids   essential fatty acids   antioxidants

nonessential amino acids   trace elements   vitamins   minerals

1. A class of substances that stabilizes free radicals   _____

2. Minerals required in very small amounts   _____

3. Complex organic molecules that are essential for metabolism   _____

4. Protein components that must be taken in as part of the diet   _____

5. Inorganic elements needed for body structure and many body functions, sometimes in large amounts   _____

6. Protein building blocks that can be manufactured by the body   _____

7. Linoleic acid is an example   _____

EXERCISE 18-6

Write the appropriate term in each blank from the list below.

zinc   iodine   iron   potassium   calcium

folate   calciferol   riboflavin   vitamin A   vitamin K

1. The vitamin that prevents dry, scaly skin and night blindness   _____

2. The vitamin needed to prevent anemia, digestive disorders, and neural tube defects in the embryo   _____

3. Another name for vitamin D, the vitamin required for normal bone formation   _____

4. The mineral component of thyroid hormones   _____

5. A mineral important in blood clotting and muscle contraction   _____

6. The characteristic element in hemoglobin, the oxygen-carrying compound in the blood   _____

7. A mineral that promotes carbon dioxide transport and energy metabolism   _____

8. A vitamin involved in the synthesis of blood clotting factors that can be synthesized by colonic bacteria   _____

8. LIST THE RECOMMENDED PERCENTAGES OF CARBOHYDRATE, FAT, AND PROTEIN IN THE DIET.

EXERCISE 18-7

Match each percentage to the corresponding nutrient type, by writing the appropriate letter in each blank.

1. protein _____   a. 55%–60%

2. fat _____   b. <30%

3. carbohydrate _____   c. 15%–20%

9. DISTINGUISH BETWEEN SIMPLE AND COMPLEX CARBOHYDRATES, GIVING EXAMPLES OF EACH.

See Exercise 18-8.

10. COMPARE SATURATED AND UNSATURATED FATS.

EXERCISE 18-8

Write the appropriate term in each blank from the list below.

trans-fatty acids   unsaturated fats   monosaccharides

saturated fats   polysaccharides   disaccharides

1. Fats that are usually of animal origin and are solid at room temperature   _____

2. Fats that are artificially saturated to prevent rancidity   _____

3. Carbohydrates with a low glycemic effect   _____

4. Glucose and fructose are examples of this type of nutrient   _____

5. Plant-derived fats that are usually liquid at room temperature _____

11. EXPLAIN HOW HEAT IS PRODUCED AND LOST IN THE BODY.

EXERCISE 18-9

Write the appropriate term in each blank from the list below.

convection   evaporation   conduction   radiation

1. The direct transfer of heat from a warmer object to a cooler one _____

2. Heat loss resulting from the conversion of a liquid, such as perspiration, to a vapor _____

3. Heat loss resulting from moving air _____

4. Heat that travels from its source as heat waves _____

12. DESCRIBE THE ROLE OF THE HYPOTHALAMUS IN REGULATING BODY TEMPERATURE.

EXERCISE 18-10

Fill in the blank after each of the following body changes—which would the hypothalamus induce when the body is cold (C), and which would it induce when the body is excessively hot (H)?

1. Constriction of the skin's blood vessels _____

2. Increased sweat gland activity _____

3. Dilation of the skin's blood vessels _____

4. Increased skeletal muscle contraction (shivering) _____

13. USING THE CASE STUDY, SUGGEST SOME DIETARY STRATEGIES FOR MANAGING HIGH BLOOD GLUCOSE LEVELS.

EXERCISE 18-11

For each of the following food choices, choose which one is healthiest and explain why. You will need to refer to information throughout the chapter.

1. whole grain bread or white bread

   _____

   _____

   _____

2. butter or olive oil

   _____

   _____

   _____

3. fruit or licorice

   _____

   _____

   _____

14. SHOW HOW WORD PARTS ARE USED TO BUILD WORDS RELATED TO METABOLISM, NUTRITION, AND BODY TEMPERATURE.

EXERCISE 18-12

Complete the following table by writing the correct word part or meaning in the space provided. Write a word that contains each word part in the Example column.

Word Part	Meaning	Example
1. -lysis	_____	_____
2. _____	sugar, sweet	_____

Making the Connections

The following concept map deals with nutrition and metabolism. Each pair of terms is linked together by a connecting phrase. Complete the concept map by filling in the appropriate term or phrase. There is one right answer for each term (1, 2, 5–7, 9, 11, 13, 14). However, there are many correct answers for the connecting phrases. Write the connecting phrases along the arrows if possible. If your phrases are too long, you may want to write them in the margins or on a separate sheet of paper.

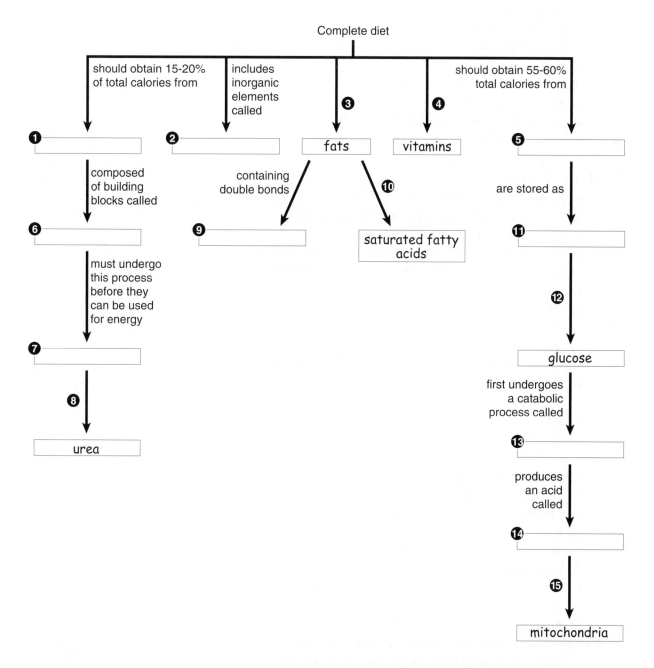

Optional Exercise: Make your own concept map, based on the regulation of body temperature. Choose your own terms to incorporate into your map, or use the following list: body temperature, dilation, constriction, hypothalamus, sweating, shivering, skin, respiratory system, radiation, convection, conduction, evaporation.

Testing Your Knowledge

BUILDING UNDERSTANDING

I. MULTIPLE CHOICE

Select the best answer and write the letter of your choice in the blank.

1. Which region of the brain is involved in temperature regulation?   1. _____
   a. hypothalamus
   b. cerebral cortex
   c. hippocampus
   d. thalamus
2. What does a complete protein contain?   2. _____
   a. all the amino acids
   b. all the essential fatty acids
   c. a variety of minerals
   d. all the essential amino acids
3. What is deamination?   3. _____
   a. an anabolic reaction
   b. the conversion of proteins into amino acids
   c. the conversion of glucose into glycogen
   d. the removal of a nitrogen group from an amino acid
4. If you have a fever, what might be your body temperature?   4. _____
   a. 96°F
   b. 39°F
   c. 39°C
   d. 96°C
5. What is the end product of the anaerobic phase of glucose catabolism?   5. _____
   a. glycogen
   b. pyruvic acid
   c. folic acid
   d. tocopherol
6. What are dietary trace elements?   6. _____
   a. sugars with a high glycemic effect
   b. vitamins needed in very small amounts
   c. minerals needed in large quantity
   d. minerals needed in very small amounts
7. Which heat transfer process is increased by profuse sweating?   7. _____
   a. radiation
   b. evaporation
   c. convection
   d. none of the above
8. Which of these phrases describes unsaturated fats?   8. _____
   a. They are generally healthier than saturated fats.
   b. They can be converted into trans fats.
   c. They contain double bonds between the carbon atoms.
   d. All of the above.

9. Which of the following is an example of an anabolic reaction?   9. _____
   a. glycerol and fatty acids are used to form a fat
   b. starches and glycogen are converted into glucose
   c. a short peptide is converted into arginine and cysteine
   d. glucose is completely oxidized to carbon dioxide and water.

II. COMPLETION EXERCISE

Write the word or phrase that correctly completes each sentence.

1. The unit used to measure energy is the _____.

2. The amount of energy needed to accomplish basic cell functions at rest is termed the _____.

3. Shivering to generate additional body heat results from increased activity of the _____.

4. Organic substances needed in small amounts in the diet are the _____.

5. The most important heat-regulating center is a section of the brain called the _____.

6. The series of catabolic reactions that results in the complete breakdown of nutrients is called _____.

7. Heat that is moved away from the skin by the wind is lost by the process of _____.

8. Glycolysis occurs in the part of the cell called the _____.

9. Fatty acids that must be consumed in the diet are called _____.

10. The only nutrient that undergoes glycolysis is _____.

UNDERSTANDING CONCEPTS

I. TRUE/FALSE

For each question, write T for true or F for false in the blank to the left of each number. If a statement is false, correct it by replacing the <u>underlined</u> term and write the correct statement in the blanks below the question.

_____ 1. A body temperature of 35°C would be considered <u>low</u>.

_____

_____ 2. Grapeseed oil is liquid at room temperature. This oil is most likely a <u>saturated</u> fat.

_____

_____ 3. The conversion of glycogen into glucose is an example of a <u>catabolic</u> reaction.

_____

_____ 4. Most heat loss in the body occurs through the <u>skin.</u>

_____

_____ 5. The element nitrogen is found in all <u>sugars.</u>

_____

_____ 6. The end product of cellular respiration in the mitochondria is <u>pyruvic acid</u>.

_____

_____ 7. The nutrient type containing the most calories per gram is <u>carbohydrate</u>.

_____

_____ 8. Copper and calcium are examples of <u>vitamins</u>.

_____

_____ 9. Linoleic acid is an example of an <u>essential amino acid</u>.

_____

II. PRACTICAL APPLICATIONS

Ms. S is researching penguin behavior at a remote location in Antarctica. She will be camping on the ice for 2 months. Study each discussion. Then write the appropriate word or phrase in the space provided.

1. Ms. S is spending her first night on the ice. She is careful to wear many layers of clothing in order to avoid a dangerous drop in body temperature. The extra clothing will reduce the transfer of heat as heat waves from her skin to the cold air. This process is called _____.

2. She is out for a moonlight walk to greet the penguins when she surprises an elephant seal stalking a penguin. Frightened, she sprints back to her tent. Her muscles are generating ATP by an oxygen-independent pathway. Each glucose molecule is generating a small number of ATP molecules, or, to be exact, _____.

3. The end product of this oxygen-independent pathway is a molecule called _____.

4. Ms. S is exercising so intensely that some of this end product is converted into a different acid. This acid, which can spill over into blood, is called _____.

5. Ms. S realizes that she lost her face mask. The howling wind results in the loss of much heat from her face by the process of _____.

6. After 2 weeks on the ice, Ms. S is out of fresh fruits and vegetables and the penguins have stolen her multivitamin supplements. She has been reading accounts of early explorers suffering from scurvy and fears she will experience the same fate. Scurvy is due to a deficiency of ascorbic acid, also known as _____.

7. Ms. S's diet is now reduced to luncheon meat and crackers. The crackers are still tasty because they contain significant amounts of artificially hydrogenated fats, known as _____.

8. She looks forward to eating her normal diet when she returns home, which is rich in complex carbohydrates, also known as _____.

III. SHORT ESSAYS

1. Is alcohol a nutrient? Defend your answer.

_____

_____

_____

_____

_____

2. A glucose molecule has been transported into a muscle cell. This cell has ample supplies of oxygen. Discuss the steps involved in using this glucose to produce energy. For each step, describe its location and oxygen requirements and name the substances produced.

_____

_____

_____

_____

_____

CONCEPTUAL THINKING

1. Your friend wants to lose some weight. She is following a diet that contains 20% carbohydrates, 40% fat, and 40% protein. Why is this diet designed to limit fat deposition? You may have to review the actions of pancreatic hormones (Chapter 11) to answer this question.

_____

_____

_____

Expanding Your Horizons

How does your diet measure up? Go to www.ChooseMyPlate.gov to find nutritional information and guidelines established by the U.S. Department of Agriculture. Some nongovernmental agencies, such as the Harvard School of Public Health, have criticized the government's efforts and proposed a graphic, the Healthy Eating Plate, that differs from the USDA guidelines. You can read about their critique at http://www.hsph.harvard.edu/nutritionsource/healthy-eating-plate/healthy-eating-plate-vs-usda-myplate/index.html (or do a Web site search for "Healthy Eating Plate").

CHAPTER 19

The Urinary System and Body Fluids

Overview

The urinary system comprises two **kidneys**, two **ureters**, one **urinary bladder**, and one **urethra**. This system is thought of as the body's main excretory mechanism; it is, in fact, often called the **excretory system.** The kidney, however, performs other essential functions; it aids in maintaining water and electrolyte balance and in regulating the acid–base balance (pH) of body fluids. The kidneys also regulate blood pressure by producing **renin,** an enzyme that activates the protein **angiotensin.** Active angiotensin increases blood pressure via actions on both the cardiovascular and the renal system.

The functional unit of the kidney is the **nephron,** which consists of a small cluster of capillaries, the **glomerulus,** and the **renal tubule.** Blood enters the glomerulus from the **afferent arteriole** and leaves via the **efferent arteriole** and subsequently passes through the **peritubular capillaries** surrounding its nephron. Water and dissolved solutes filter from blood in the glomerulus into the proximal portion of the renal tubule, the **glomerular capsule.** The resulting fluid (the filtrate) passes through the rest of the renal tubule—the proximal tubule, nephron loop, and distal tubule—before entering the **collecting duct** and draining into the renal pelvis as **urine.** The filtrate is substantially modified as it passes through the renal tubule. Most of the water and solutes return to the bloodstream by the process of **reabsorption;** some solutes pass from peritubular blood into the tubule by the process of **secretion.** Finally, under the influence of antidiuretic hormone (ADH), the tubular fluid is concentrated just enough to maintain normal body fluid balance.

The majority (50% to 70%) of a person's body weight is **water.** This water is a solvent, a transport medium, and a participant in metabolic reactions. A variety of substances are dissolved in this water, including electrolytes, nutrients, gases, enzymes, hormones, and waste products. Body fluids are distributed in two main compartments: (1) the **intracellular fluid** compartment within the cells and (2) the **extracellular fluid** compartment located outside the cells. The latter category includes blood plasma, interstitial fluid separating cells, lymph, and fluids in special compartments, such as the humors of the eye, cerebrospinal fluid, serous fluids, and synovial fluids.

Water balance is maintained by matching fluid intake with fluid output. Fluid intake is stimulated by the thirst center in the **hypothalamus,** but humans voluntarily control their fluid intake and may consume excess or insufficient fluids. Normally, the amount of fluid taken in with food and beverages equals the amount of fluid lost through the skin and the respiratory, digestive, and urinary tracts.

The composition of intracellular and extracellular fluids is an important factor in homeostasis. These fluids must have the proper levels of electrolytes and must be kept at a constant pH. The kidneys are the main regulators of body fluids. They alter the retention of specific electrolytes and water in response to hormones such as aldosterone, antidiuretic hormone (ADH), atrial natriuretic peptide (ANP), and parathyroid hormone. Buffers and the respiratory system aid the kidneys in maintaining constant blood pH. The normal pH of body fluids is a slightly alkaline 7.4.

Addressing the Learning Outcomes

1. DESCRIBE THE ORGANS OF THE URINARY SYSTEM AND GIVE THE FUNCTIONS OF EACH.

EXERCISE 19-1: Male Urinary System (Text Fig. 19-1)

1. Write the name of each structure in the line next to the bullet. (Hint: Structure 1 carries oxygen-rich blood).
2. If you wish, color arteries red, veins blue, and structures encountering urine yellow.
3. Put arrows in the small boxes to indicate the direction of blood/urine movement.

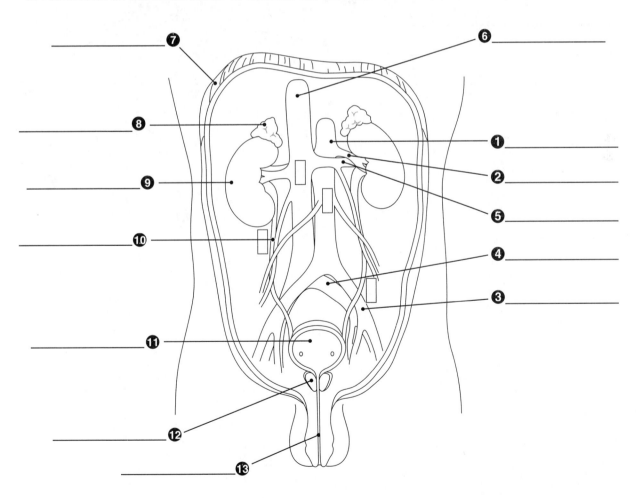

EXERCISE 19-2: Kidney Structure and the Renal Blood Supply (Text Fig. 19-2)

1. Write the names of the blood vessels on lines 1 and 2 (vessel 1 drains from the abdominal aorta and vessel 2 drains into the inferior vena cava). Use red for the artery and blue for the vein.
2. Color the artery and arterioles on the diagram red and the veins and venules blue.
3. Write the names of the remaining structures on the appropriate numbered lines in different colors, and color the structures on the diagram. Use the same, dark color for structures 3 and 4. Use the same color for structures 6 and 7. Use yellow for structures 8 to 10.

1. _____

2. _____

3. _____

4. _____

5. _____

6. _____

7. _____

8. _____

9. _____

10. _____

EXERCISE 19-3

Write the appropriate term in each blank from the list below.

ureter   urinary bladder   urethra   renal capsule   renal cortex

retroperitoneal space   nephron   renal pelvis   adipose capsule   renal medulla

1. A funnel-shaped basin that collects urine from collecting ducts   _____

2. The tube that carries urine from the bladder to the outside   _____

3. The area behind the peritoneum that contains the ureters
   and the kidneys   _____

4. A microscopic functional unit of the kidney   _____

5. A tube connecting a kidney with the bladder   _____

6. The crescent of fat that helps to support the kidney   _____

7. The inner region of the kidney   _____

8. The outer region of the kidney   _____

2. LIST THE SYSTEMS THAT ELIMINATE WASTE AND NAME THE SUBSTANCES ELIMINATED BY EACH.

EXERCISE 19-4

For each substance, determine the system or systems that eliminate it and write the appropriate letter(s) in the blank (U for urinary, D for digestive, R for respiratory, and I for integumentary). There may be more than one answer for each substance.

1. Carbon dioxide _____

2. Bile _____

3. Water _____

4. Salts _____

5. Digestive residue _____

6. Nitrogenous wastes _____

3. LIST THE ACTIVITIES OF THE KIDNEYS IN MAINTAINING HOMEOSTASIS.

EXERCISE 19-5

In the spaces below, list five body parameters that the kidney helps to maintain within tight limits.

1. _____
2. _____
3. _____
4. _____
5. _____

4. TRACE THE PATH OF A DROP OF BLOOD AS IT FLOWS THROUGH THE KIDNEY.

See Exercises 19-6 and 19-7.

5. DESCRIBE A NEPHRON.

EXERCISE 19-6: A Nephron and Its Blood Supply (Text Fig. 19-3)

1. Follow the passage of blood by labeling structures 1 to 6. Use different shades of red for the arteries/arterioles, purple for the capillaries, and blue for the venules/veins. Lines indicate the boundaries between different vessels.
2. Follow the passage of filtrate through the nephron by labeling structures 7 to 13. Use different colors (perhaps shades of yellow and orange) for the different structures. Lines indicate the boundaries between the different nephron parts.
3. Write the names of the remaining structures on the appropriate numbered lines in different colors, and color the structures on the diagram. Bullets 14 and 15 indicate the two major divisions of the kidney.

1. _____
2. _____
3. _____
4. _____
5. _____
6. _____
7. _____
8. _____
9. _____
10. _____
11. _____
12. _____
13. _____
14. _____
15. _____

EXERCISE 19-7

Write the appropriate term in each blank from the list below.

afferent arteriole   proximal tubule   peritubular capillaries   nephron loop
glomerulus   glomerular capsule   efferent arteriole   renal artery
renal vein   collecting duct

1. A hollow bulb at the proximal end of the renal tubule   _____

2. The blood vessels connecting the afferent and efferent arterioles _____

3. The portion of the nephron receiving filtrate from the glomerular capsule   _____

4. The vessel that branches to form the glomerulus   _____

5. The vessel that drains the kidney   _____

6. The blood vessels that exchange substances with the nephron   _____

7. A tube that receives urine from the distal tubule   _____

8. The portion of the nephron that dips into the medulla   _____

6. NAME THE FOUR PROCESSES INVOLVED IN URINE FORMATION AND DESCRIBE THE ACTION OF EACH.

EXERCISE 19-8: Glomerular Filtration (Text Fig. 19-5)

1. Write the names of the different structures on the appropriate numbered lines in different colors, and lightly shade the structures on the diagram. Use different shades of red for structures 1 to 3, and yellow for part 7. Do not color over the symbols. Some structures have appeared on earlier diagrams. You may want to use the same color scheme.

2. Color the symbols beside "soluble molecules," "proteins," and "blood cells" in different, dark colors and color the corresponding symbols on the diagram.

1. _____

2. _____

3. _____

4. _____

5. _____

6. _____

7. _____

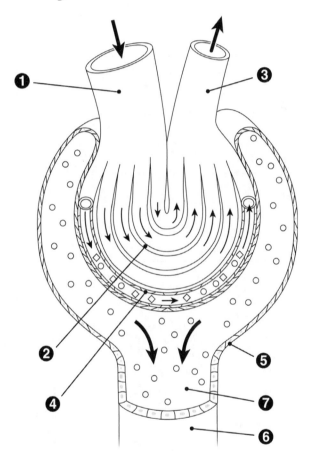

○ Soluble molecules
◇ Proteins
○ Blood cells

EXERCISE 19-9: Summary of Urine Formation (Text Fig. 19-7)

1. Label the structures and fluids by writing the appropriate terms on lines 5 to 11.
2. Write the name the hormone that controls water reabsorption in the collecting duct on line 12.
3. Write and briefly describe the different kidney processes in lines 1 to 4.

1. _____

2. _____

3. _____

4. _____

5. _____

6. _____

7. _____

8. _____

9. _____

10. _____

11. _____

12. _____

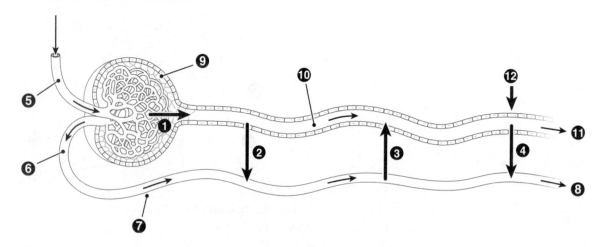

7. IDENTIFY HORMONES INVOLVED IN URINE FORMATION AND CITE THE FUNCTION OF EACH.

EXERCISE 19-10

Match the substances to their description/action by writing the appropriate letter in each blank. Letters can be used more than once or not at all.

_____ 1. Directly increases sodium reabsorption   a. aldosterone

_____ 2. Acts on the glomerular capsule to increase filtration   b. atrial natriuretic peptide

_____ 3. Synthesized in the hypothalamus   c. antidiuretic hormone

_____ 4. An enzyme   d. renin

_____ 5. Acts to reduce blood pressure   e. angiotensin

_____ 6. Directly promotes urine concentration   f. none of the above

_____ 7. Stimulates blood vessel constriction *and* water retention

8. DESCRIBE THE COMPONENTS AND FUNCTIONS OF THE JUXTAGLOMERULAR (JG) APPARATUS.

EXERCISE 19-11: The Juxtaglomerular (JG) Apparatus (Text Fig. 19-8)

Write the names of the different structures on the appropriate numbered lines in different colors, and color the structures on the diagram. Use different shades of red for structures 1 to 3. (Hint: Blood flows from structure 1 toward structure 2). Use a dark color for structure 8. Some structures have appeared on earlier diagrams. You may want to use the same color scheme.

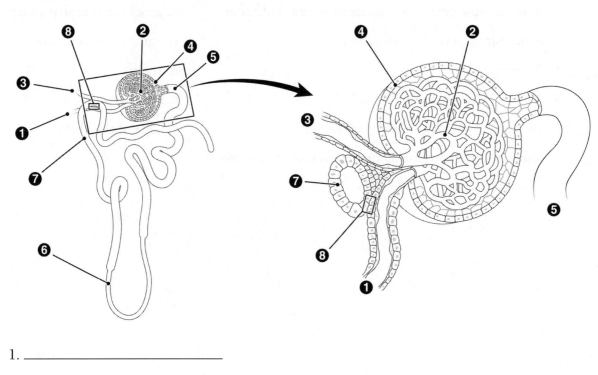

1. _____

2. _____

3. _____

4. _____

5. _____

6. _____

7. _____

8. _____

EXERCISE 19-12

Write the appropriate term in each blank from the list below.

renin   juxtaglomerular apparatus   urea   EPO
filtration   tubular reabsorption   tubular secretion   antidiuretic hormone
angiotensin   aldosterone

1. An enzyme produced by the kidney _____

2. The hormone that increases sodium reabsorption in the distal tubule _____

3. The process that returns useful substances in the filtrate to the bloodstream _____

4. The process by which substances leave the glomerulus and enter the glomerular capsule _____

5. The structure in the kidney that produces renin _____

6. The hormone produced in the kidney that stimulates erythrocyte production by the bone marrow _____

7. The process by which the renal tubule actively moves substances from the blood into the nephron to be excreted _____

8. The hormone that increases the permeability of the collecting duct to water _____

9. DESCRIBE THE PROCESS OF MICTURITION.

EXERCISE 19-13: The Male Urinary Bladder (Text Fig. 19-9)

Label the indicated parts. Hint: Bullet 3 labels "wrinkles" in the bladder wall.

1. _____
2. _____
3. _____
4. _____
5. _____
6. _____
7. _____
8. _____
9. _____

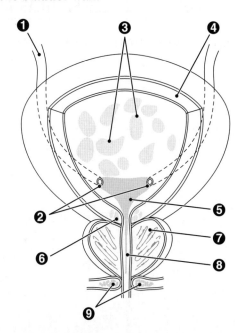

EXERCISE 19-14

Label each of the following statements as true (T) or false (F).

1. The internal urethral sphincter is formed of skeletal muscle.   _____

2. The external urethral sphincter is formed by the pelvic floor muscles.   _____

3. When the bladder fills with liquid, stretch receptors are activated.   _____

4. When the bladder fills with liquid, muscles in the bladder wall contract.   _____

5. Urination will occur when the external urethral sphincter is contracted.   _____

10. NAME THREE NORMAL CONSTITUENTS OF URINE.

EXERCISE 19-15

Circle the three constituents you would expect to find in normal urine.

1. Glucose

2. Blood

3. Pigment

4. Nitrogenous waste products

5. White blood cells

6. Electrolytes

11. COMPARE INTRACELLULAR AND EXTRACELLULAR FLUIDS.

See Exercises 19-16 to 19-18.

12. LIST FOUR TYPES OF EXTRACELLULAR FLUIDS.

EXERCISE 19-16: Main Fluid Compartments (Text Fig. 19-10)

Label the different fluid compartments.

1. _____

2. _____

3. _____

4. _____

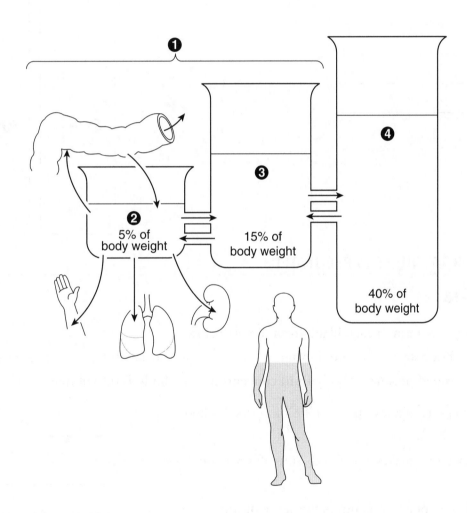

13. NAME THE SYSTEMS THAT ARE INVOLVED IN WATER BALANCE.

EXERCISE 19-17: Daily Gain and Loss of Water (Text Fig. 19-11)

Write the names of the different sources of water gain and loss on the appropriate numbered lines in different colors. Color the diagram with the appropriate colors.

1. _____
2. _____
3. _____
4. _____
5. _____
6. _____
7. _____

Water gain 2500 mL/day | Water loss 2500 mL/day

❶ 200 mL | ❹ 200 mL
❷ 700 mL | ❺ 300 mL
         | ❻ 500 mL
❸ 1600 mL | ❼ 1500 mL

14. EXPLAIN HOW THIRST IS REGULATED.

EXERCISE 19-18

Write the appropriate term in each blank from the list below.

hypothalamus   brainstem   interstitial   intracellular   extracellular
water   blood plasma   body fluid concentration   body fluid volume

1. The substance that makes up about 4% of a person's body weight _____

2. The substance that makes up 50% to 70% of a person's body weight _____

3. The part of the brain that controls the sense of thirst _____

4. Term that specifically describes fluids in the microscopic spaces between cells _____

5. The thirst center is stimulated when this is increased _____

6. The thirst center is stimulated when this is decreased _____

7. Term that describes the fluid within the body cells _____

15. DEFINE *ELECTROLYTES* AND DESCRIBE SOME OF THEIR FUNCTIONS.

EXERCISE 19-19

Write the appropriate term in each blank from the list below.

cation   anion   potassium   phosphate

electrolyte   sodium   calcium   chloride

1. A general term describing any positively charged ion   _____

2. A general term describing any negatively charged ion   _____

3. A component of stomach acid   _____

4. The most abundant cation inside cells   _____

5. A compound that forms ions in solution   _____

6. A cation involved in bone formation   _____

7. The most abundant cation in the fluid surrounding cells   _____

16. DESCRIBE THE ROLE OF HORMONES IN ELECTROLYTE BALANCE.

EXERCISE 19-20

Write the appropriate term in each blank from the list below.

parathyroid hormone   antidiuretic hormone

atrial natriuretic peptide   aldosterone

1. A hormone secreted from the posterior pituitary that causes the kidney to reabsorb water   _____

2. A hormone that is secreted when blood pressure rises too high   _____

3. The adrenal hormone that promotes sodium reabsorption by the kidney   _____

4. A hormone that causes the kidney to reabsorb calcium   _____

17. DESCRIBE THREE METHODS FOR REGULATING THE pH OF BODY FLUIDS.

EXERCISE 19-21

Write the appropriate term in each blank below and on the next page from the list below.

buffer   hydrogen ion   kidney   lung   carbon dioxide

1. Any substance that aids in maintaining a constant pH   _____

2. The substance that directly determines the acidity or alkalinity of a fluid   _____

3. The organ that regulates pH balance by altering urine acidity   _____

4. The organ that regulates pH balance by altering carbon dioxide retention   _____

18. REFERRING TO THE CASE STUDY, DESCRIBE HOW URETHRAL BLOCKAGE CAN AFFECT KIDNEY FUNCTION.

EXERCISE 19-22

Fill in the blanks in the following description. Refer to the case study in your textbook if required.

Adam was suffering from the enlargement of his (1) _____ gland, a doughnut-shaped structure inferior to his urinary bladder. When Adam attempted to urinate, a process described as (2) _____, he voluntarily relaxed his (3) _____ _____ sphincter. However, urine did not readily flow because his enlarged gland restricted flow through the (4) _____. He was unable to void his urinary bladder, and urine backed up and distended the (5) _____, which carry urine to the bladder. This distention is called (6) _____. Urine further backed up into his kidneys, causing (7) _____, or "water in the kidneys." Adam's urologist diagnosed his enlarged prostate using an instrument called a(n) (8) _____ and removed pieces of his prostate using an instrument called a(n) (9) _____.

19. SHOW HOW WORD PARTS ARE USED TO BUILD WORDS RELATED TO THE URINARY SYSTEM AND BODY FLUIDS.

EXERCISE 19-23

Complete the following table by writing the correct word part or meaning in the space provided. Write a word that contains each word part in the Example column.

Word Part	Meaning	Example
1. _____	night	_____
2. extra-	_____	_____
3. _____	many	_____
4. semi-	_____	_____
5. nephr/o	_____	_____
6. _____	within	_____
7. _____	backward, behind	_____
8. _____	next to	_____
9. ren/o	_____	_____
10. osmo-	_____	_____

Making the Connections

The following concept map deals with the organization of the kidney. Each pair of terms is linked together by a connecting phrase into a sentence. Complete the concept map by filling in the appropriate term or phrase. There is one right answer for each term. However, there are many correct answers for the connecting phrases (2, 3, 6). Bullets 12 through 15 refer to the four processes of urine formation. Figure out which bullet refers to which process.

Map A

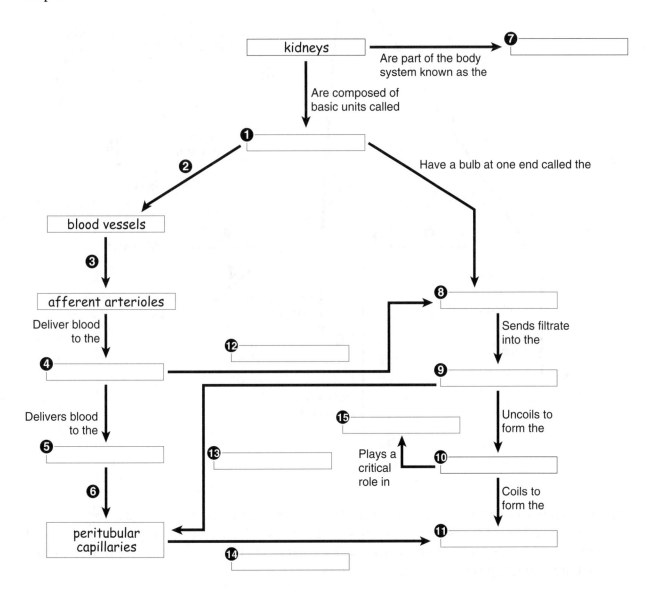

Map B

The following concept map deals with the types of body fluids and the sources of fluid input and output. Each pair of terms is linked together by a connecting phrase. Complete the concept map by filling in the appropriate term or phrase. There is one right answer for each term. However, there are many correct answers for the connecting phrases (4–7, 9, 11, 14, 15).

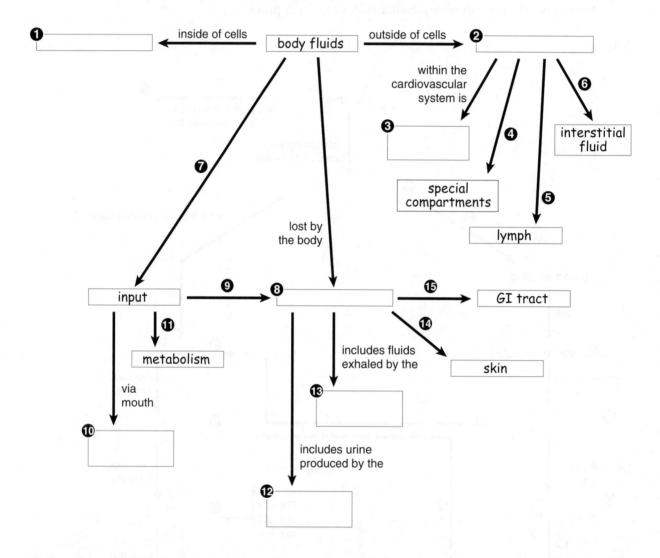

Optional Exercise: Choose your own terms to incorporate into your map, or use the following list: Urinary system, kidneys, nephrons, ureters, urinary bladder, urethra, adipose capsule, renal capsule, renal pelvis, rugae, trigone, urinary meatus, penis, micturition, internal urethral sphincter, external urethral sphincter.

Testing Your Knowledge

BUILDING UNDERSTANDING

I. MULTIPLE CHOICE

Select the best answer and write the letter of your choice in the blank.

1. What is the correct order of urine flow from its source to the outside
   of the body?   1. _____
   a. urethra, bladder, kidney, ureter
   b. bladder, kidney, urethra, ureter
   c. kidney, ureter, bladder, urethra
   d. kidney, urethra, bladder, ureter

2. What is the correct order of filtrate flow through the nephron?   2. _____
   a. nephron loop, distal tubule, proximal tubule, collecting duct
   b. glomerular capsule, proximal tubule, nephron loop, distal tubule
   c. proximal tubule, distal tubule, nephron loop, glomerular capsule
   d. glomerular capsule, distal tubule, proximal tubule, collecting duct

3. Which of the following substances reduces blood pressure?   3. _____
   a. aldosterone
   b. antidiuretic hormone
   c. atrial natriuretic peptide
   d. angiotensin

4. The juxtaglomerular apparatus consists of cells in what areas?   4. _____
   a. proximal tubule and efferent arteriole
   b. renal artery and afferent arteriole
   c. collecting tubules and renal vein
   d. distal tubule and afferent arteriole

5. Which of the following is NOT a function of the kidneys?   5. _____
   a. red blood cell destruction
   b. blood pressure regulation
   c. elimination of nitrogenous wastes
   d. modification of body fluid composition

6. Which of these processes moves substances from the distal tubule to
   the peritubular capillaries?   6. _____
   a. secretion
   b. filtration
   c. reabsorption
   d. excretion

7. Which of these substances would *not* be found in normal urine?   7. _____
   a. sodium
   b. hydrogen
   c. red blood cells
   d. urea

8. Which of these terms describes the process of expelling urine?   8. _____
   a. reabsorption
   b. micturition
   c. dehydration
   d. defecation

9. Which of these terms describes the indentation where the blood
   vessels and ureter attaches to the kidney?   9. _____
   a. renal pyramid
   b. hilum
   c. calyx
   d. ptosis

10. Which of these structures produces aldosterone?   10. _____
    a. hypothalamus
    b. pituitary
    c. kidney
    d. adrenal cortex

11. Which of these is an action of antidiuretic hormone?   11. _____
    a. increases salt excretion by the kidney
    b. inhibits thirst
    c. decreases urine output
    d. increases calcium reabsorption by the kidney

12. Which minerals are required for normal bone formation?   12. _____
    a. calcium
    b. phosphate
    c. neither calcium nor phosphate
    d. both calcium and phosphate

13. Which of the following is NOT a buffer?   13. _____
    a. hemoglobin
    b. bicarbonate
    c. oxygen
    d. phosphate

14. Which of the following fluids is NOT in the extracellular
    compartment?   14. _____
    a. cytoplasm
    b. cerebrospinal fluid
    c. lymph
    d. interstitial fluid

II. COMPLETION EXERCISE

Write the word or phrase that correctly completes each sentence.

1. A negatively charged ion is called a(n) _____.

2. The receptors that detect an increase in body fluid concentration are called

_____.

3. The ion that plays the largest role in maintaining body fluid volume is

_____.

4. When the bladder is empty, its lining is thrown into the folds known as

_____.

5. The vessel that brings blood to the glomerulus is the _____.

6. Water balance is partly regulated by a thirst center located in a region of the brain called the

_____.

7. The distal tubule empties its fluid into the _____.

8. The hormone that decreases blood volume is _____.

9. Fluid passes from capillaries into the glomerular capsule of the nephron by the process of

_____.

10. The capillaries involved in filtration are called the _____.

11. The capillaries that surround the nephron are called the _____.

UNDERSTANDING CONCEPTS

I. TRUE/FALSE

For each question, write T for true or F for false in the blank to the left of each number. If a statement is false, correct it by replacing the underlined term and write the correct statement in the blanks below the question.

_____ 1. Excessive water loss in the urine could be caused by a deficiency of the hypothalamic hormone erythropoietin.

_____

_____ 2. The movement of hydrogen ions from the peritubular capillaries into the distal tubule is an example of tubular secretion.

_____

_____ 3. The exhalation of carbon dioxide makes the blood more acidic.

_____

_____ 4. Urine with a specific gravity of 0.05 is <u>more</u> concentrated than urine with a specific gravity of 0.04.

_____

_____ 5. Aldosterone tends to <u>decrease</u> the amount of urine produced.

_____

_____ 6. Voluntary control of urination involves the <u>internal</u> urethral sphincter.

_____

_____ 7. The triangular-shaped region in the floor of the bladder is called the <u>renal pelvis.</u>

_____

_____ 8. Most water loss occurs through the actions of the <u>digestive</u> system.

_____

_____ 9. The fluids found in joint capsules and in the eyeball are examples of <u>extracellular fluids</u>.

_____

_____ 10. The organ that excretes the largest amount of water per day is the <u>skin.</u>

_____

II. PRACTICAL APPLICATIONS

Study each discussion. Then write the appropriate word or phrase in the space provided.

➤ Group A

1. Ms. S, age 26, was teaching English in rural India. She developed severe diarrhea, probably as a result of a questionable pakora from a road-side stand. On admission to a hospital, she was found to be seriously dehydrated. Ms. S's blood will contain high levels of a hormone synthesized by the hypothalamus called _____.

2. The physician's first concern was to increase Ms. S's plasma volume. Her fluid deficit was addressed by administering a 0.9% sodium chloride solution. This solution contains the same concentration of solutes as Ms. S's cells and is thus termed _____.

3. Next a nurse assistant tested the pH of Ms. S's blood. The normal pH range of blood is _____.

4. Ms. S's blood pH was found to be abnormal, and sodium bicarbonate was added to her IV. Bicarbonate is an example of a substance that helps maintain a constant pH. These substances are known as _____.

➤ **Group B**

1. Young S, aged 1, was brought to the hospital with an enlarged abdomen. His blood pressure was shown to be extremely high, a disorder that can result from increased renin production. Renin is produced by a specialized region of the kidney called the _____.

2. S was administered a medication that blocks renin action. Renin normally activates a substance called _____.

3. Further testing showed that S was suffering from the irreversible loss of the small units of the kidney that produce urine. These units are the _____.

4. S's enlarged abdomen resulted from the accumulation of fluid between cells. This type of fluid is most accurately described as _____.

5. S was also quite lethargic, due to a deficiency in red blood cells. This deficiency probably reflects the fact that the kidney synthesizes a hormone called _____.

III. SHORT ESSAYS

1. Compare and contrast the processes of filtration and secretion. Name at least one similarity and two differences.

_____

_____

_____

_____

_____

2. Explain why breath holding will increase blood acidity, and how the kidney would respond to repeated episodes of breath holding.

_____

_____

_____

_____

_____

CONCEPTUAL THINKING

1. Ms. W has just eaten a large bag of salty popcorn. Her blood is now too salty and must be diluted. Is it possible for the kidney to increase water reabsorption without increasing salt absorption? Explain.

   _____

   _____

   _____

   _____

2. Mr. R is taking penicillin to cure a throat infection. He must take the drug frequently because the kidney clears penicillin very efficiently. That is, all of the penicillin that enters the renal artery leaves the kidney in the urine. However, only some penicillin molecules will be filtered into the glomerular capsule. How can the kidney excrete all of the penicillin it receives?

   _____

   _____

   _____

   _____

3. Ms. J is stranded on a desert island with limited water supplies. A. How will the volume and concentration of her body fluids change? B. How will her hypothalamus and pituitary gland respond to these changes? C. What will be the net effect of these responses?

   _____

   _____

   _____

4. Your summer research project is to design new drugs to alter blood pressure by altering water retention and thus blood volume. You know that increasing blood volume increases blood pressure and vice versa. You test three different compounds, listed below. Predict the effect of each compound on blood pressure, and defend your answer.

(Note: Agonists mimic the effect of the hormone, and antagonists block the effect of the hormone).

a. a parathyroid hormone agonist

_____

_____

_____

b. an aldosterone antagonist

_____

_____

_____

c. an atrial natriuretic peptide (ANP) agonist

_____

_____

_____

Expanding Your Horizons

How much salt do you eat in a day? The average American consumes far more salt than the recommended 1100 to 3300 mg/d. One frozen entree, for instance, can contain 700 mg of salt or more! Track your salt intake over a few days, and see how you compare. Use the nutritional labels on prepared foods and this Web site below to gauge the sodium content of different foods.

- USDA National Nutrient Database for Standard Reference, Release 17. Available at http://www.nal.usda.gov/fnic/foodcomp/Data/SR17/wtrank/sr17a307.pdf

Perpetuation of Life

CHAPTER

20

The Male and Female Reproductive Systems

Overview

Reproduction is the process by which life continues. Human reproduction is **sexual**; that is, it requires the union of two different *germ cells* or **gametes**. (Some simple forms of life can reproduce without a partner in the process of **asexual** reproduction.) These germ cells, the **spermatozoon** in males and the **ovum** in females, are formed by **meiosis**, a type of cell division in which the chromosome number is reduced by half. When fertilization occurs and the gametes combine, the original chromosome number is restored.

The **gonads** manufacture the gametes and also produce hormones. These activities are continuous in the male but cyclic in the female. The male gonad is the **testis**. The remainder of the male reproductive tract consists of passageways for storage and transport of spermatozoa; the male organ of copulation, the **penis**; and several glands that contribute to the production of **semen**.

The female gonad is the **ovary**. The ovum released each month at the time of **ovulation** travels through the **uterine tubes** to the **uterus**, where the ovum, if fertilized, develops. If no fertilization occurs, the ovum, along with the built-up lining of the uterus, is eliminated through the **vagina** as the **menstrual flow**.

Reproduction is under the control of hormones from the **anterior pituitary**, which, in turn, is controlled by the **hypothalamus** of the brain. These organs respond to **feedback** mechanisms, which maintain proper hormone levels.

Aging causes changes in both the male and female reproductive systems. A gradual decrease in male hormone production begins as early as age 20 and continues throughout life. In the female, a more sudden decrease in activity occurs between ages 45 and 55 and ends in **menopause**, the cessation of menstruation and of the childbearing years.

Addressing the Learning Outcomes

1. IDENTIFY THE MALE AND FEMALE GAMETES AND STATE THE PURPOSE OF MEIOSIS.

EXERCISE 20-1

Label each of the following statements as true (T) or false (F). Exercise 20-4 relates to the male and female gametes.

1. Meiosis occurs only in germ cells. _____

2. The cells formed by meiosis have the same number of
   chromosomes as the parent cell. _____

2. NAME THE GONADS AND ACCESSORY ORGANS OF THE MALE REPRODUCTIVE SYSTEM AND CITE THE FUNCTION OF EACH.

EXERCISE 20-2: Male Reproductive System (Text Fig. 20-1A)

1. Write the names of the structures that are not part of the reproductive system on the appropriate lines 1 to 6 in different colors. Use the same color for structures 1 and 2 and for structures 4 and 5. Color the structures on the diagram.
2. Write the names of the parts of the male reproductive system on the appropriate lines 7 to 20 in different colors. Use the same color for structures 10 and 11. Color the structures on the diagram.

1. _____
2. _____
3. _____
4. _____
5. _____
6. _____
7. _____
8. _____
9. _____
10. _____
11. _____
12. _____
13. _____
14. _____
15. _____
16. _____
17. _____
18. _____
19. _____
20. _____

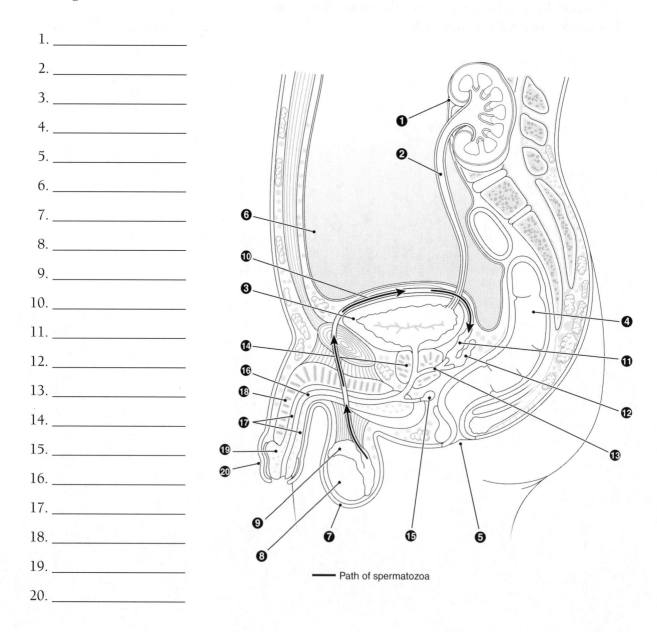

Path of spermatozoa

EXERCISE 20-3: Structure of the Testis (Text Fig. 20-1B)

Label the indicated parts. (Hint: the vein is more branched than the artery).

1. _____
2. _____
3. _____
4. _____
5. _____
6. _____
7. _____
8. _____
9. _____
10. _____
11. _____
12. _____

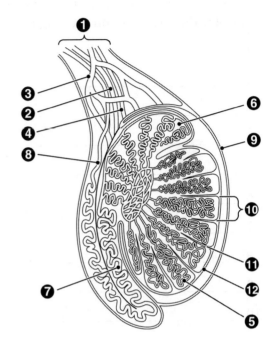

EXERCISE 20-4

Write the appropriate term in each blank from the list below.

interstitial cell   sustentacular cell spermatozoon ovum

seminiferous tubule   ovarian follicle

1. A cell that nourishes and protects developing spermatozoa   _____

2. A cell that secretes testosterone   _____

3. The male gamete   _____

4. The female gamete   _____

5. The cluster of cells that surrounds the female gamete   _____

EXERCISE 20-5: Cross Section of the Penis (Text Fig. 20-5)

1. Write the names of the parts on the appropriate lines in different colors. (Hint: the nerve is solid and the veins have larger lumens).
2. Color the structures on the diagram.

1. _____

2. _____

3. _____

4. _____

5. _____

6. _____

7. _____

8. _____

9. _____

10. _____

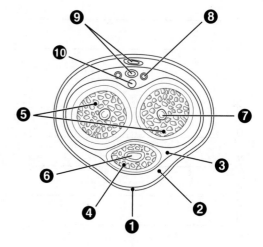

3. DESCRIBE THE COMPOSITION AND FUNCTION OF SEMEN.

EXERCISE 20-6

In the spaces below, list five functions of semen.

1. _____

2. _____

3. _____

4. _____

5. _____

4. DRAW AND LABEL A SPERMATOZOON.

EXERCISE 20-7: Diagram of a Human Spermatozoon (Text Fig. 20-4)

1. Write the names of the parts on the appropriate lines in different colors. Use black for structures 1 to 3 because they will not be colored.
2. Color the structures on the diagram.

1. _____

2. _____

3. _____

4. _____

5. _____

6. _____

7. _____

5. IDENTIFY THE TWO HORMONES THAT REGULATE THE PRODUCTION AND DEVELOPMENT OF THE MALE GAMETES.

EXERCISE 20-8

Write the name of the appropriate hormone in each blank. Each hormone may be used more than once. Note that questions 1 and 5 have *two* blanks because the statement applies to *two* hormones.

testosterone   **luteinizing hormone**   **follicle-stimulating hormone**

1. Produced by the anterior pituitary gland   _____

2. Produced by the testicular interstitial cells   _____

3. Stimulates testicular interstitial cells   _____

4. Stimulates testosterone production   _____

5. Stimulates the formation and development of spermatozoa   _____

6. Directly stimulates the development of secondary sex
   characteristics   _____

7. Stimulates sustentacular cells   _____

6. NAME THE GONADS AND ACCESSORY ORGANS OF THE FEMALE REPRODUCTIVE SYSTEM AND CITE THE FUNCTION OF EACH.

EXERCISE 20-9: Female Reproductive System (Text Fig. 20-6)

1. Write the names of the parts on the appropriate lines in different colors. Use the same color for parts 8 and 9, for parts 10 to 13, and for parts 14 and 15.
2. Color the structures on the diagram.

1. _____

2. _____

3. _____

4. _____

5. _____

6. _____

7. _____

8. _____

9. _____

10. _____

11. _____

12. _____

13. _____

14. _____

15. _____

16. _____

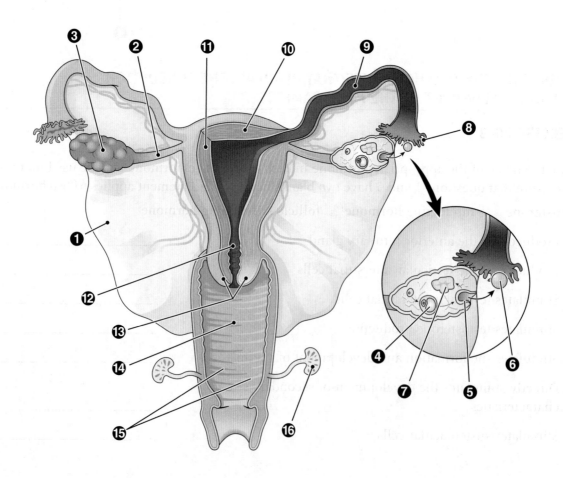

EXERCISE 20-10: Female Reproductive System (Sagittal Section) (Text Fig. 20-9)

1. Write the names of the structures that are not part of the reproductive system on the appropriate lines 1 to 8 in different colors. Use the same color for structures 1 and 2, for structures 3 and 4, and for structures 5 and 6. Color the structures on the diagram.
2. Write the names of the parts of the female reproductive system and supporting ligaments on the appropriate lines 9 to 19 in different colors. Use the same color for structures 15 and 16. Color the structures on the diagram.

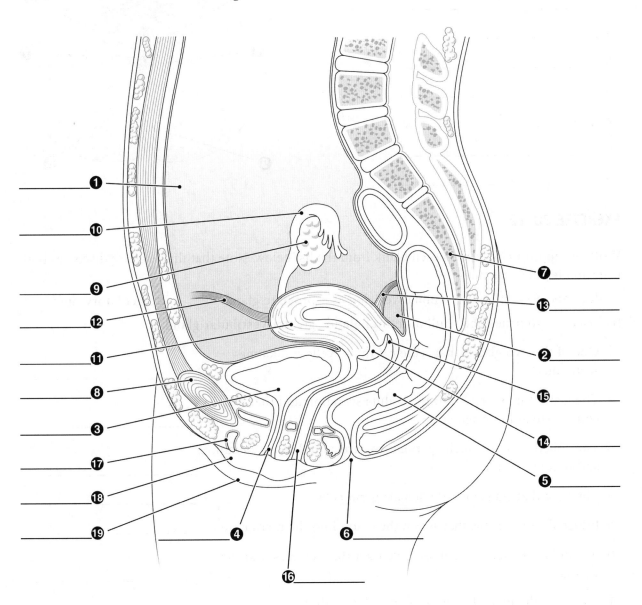

EXERCISE 20-11: External Parts of the Female Reproductive System (Text Fig. 20-10)

Label the indicated parts.

1. _____
2. _____
3. _____
4. _____
5. _____
6. _____
7. _____
8. _____
9. _____

EXERCISE 20-12

Write the appropriate term in each blank from the list below. Note that this exercise discusses both male and female structures.

epididymis   vas deferens   seminal vesicle   prostate gland   ejaculatory duct
fimbriae   uterine tube   bulbourethral gland   greater vestibular gland

1. One of the two glands that secrete a thick, yellow, alkaline secretion _____

2. The gland that secretes a thin alkaline secretion and that can contract to aid in ejaculation _____

3. The coiled tube in which spermatozoa are stored as they mature and become motile _____

4. The tube that transports the female germ cells _____

5. Fringelike extensions that sweep the ovum into the uterine tube _____

6. A gland in the female reproductive tract that secretes into the vagina _____

7. A duct in the male that empties into the urethra _____

8. A gland located inferior to the prostate that secretes mucus during sexual stimulation _____

EXERCISE 20-13

Write the appropriate term in each blank from the list below.

cervix   myometrium   fundus   vestibule

endometrium   fornix   hymen   perineum

1. The Bartholin glands secrete into this area   _____

2. The vaginal region around the cervix   _____

3. The specialized tissue that lines the uterus   _____

4. The small, rounded part of the uterus located above the
openings of the uterine tubes   _____

5. A fold of membrane found at the opening of the vagina   _____

6. The necklike part of the uterus that dips into the upper vagina   _____

7. The muscular wall of the uterus   _____

7. LIST IN THE CORRECT ORDER THE HORMONES PRODUCED DURING THE MENSTRUAL CYCLE AND CITE THE SOURCE OF EACH.

EXERCISE 20-14: The Menstrual Cycle (Text Fig. 20-11)

1. Identify the hormone responsible for each of the numbered lines (bullets 1 to 4), and write the hormone names on the appropriate lines in different colors. Trace over the lines in the graph with the appropriate color.
2. Write the names of the phases of the ovarian cycle (bullets 5, 6, and 9) and the uterine cycle (bullets 7, 8 and 10) on the appropriate lines.

1. _____

2. _____

3. _____

4. _____

5. _____

6. _____

7. _____

8. _____

9. _____

10. _____

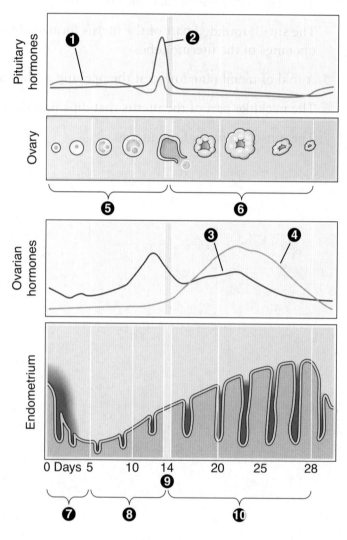

EXERCISE 20-15

Write the appropriate term in each blank from the list below.

luteinizing hormone   follicle-stimulating hormone   estrogen   progesterone

corpus luteum   ovulation   menstruation

1. A hormone that is produced only during the luteal phase of the menstrual cycle

   _____

2. An ovarian hormone that is produced during the follicular and luteal phases of the menstrual cycle

   _____

3. Discharge of an ovum from the surface of the ovary

   _____

4. The hormone that stimulates the development of the cells surrounding the ovum

   _____

5. The structure formed by the ruptured follicle after ovulation   _____

6. The phase of the menstrual cycle when the endometrium is degenerating

   _____

8. DESCRIBE THE CHANGES THAT OCCUR DURING AND AFTER MENOPAUSE.

EXERCISE 20-16

In the spaces below, write five different changes that may be associated with menopause.

1. _____

2. _____

3. _____

4. _____

5. _____

9. CITE THE MAIN METHODS OF BIRTH CONTROL IN USE.

EXERCISE 20-17

Write the appropriate term in each blank from the list below.

IUD   birth control patch   birth control ring   vasectomy   tubal ligation
male condom   diaphragm

1. A method used to administer estrogen and progesterone through the skin   _____

2. A device implanted into the uterus that prevents fertilization and implantation   _____

3. A rubber cap fitted over the cervix   _____

4. The birth control method that is also highly effective against sexually transmitted infections   _____

5. A method used to administer birth control hormones internally   _____

6. A surgical method of birth control in females   _____

10. REFERRING TO THE CASE STUDY, DISCUSS SOME PROCEDURES USED TO DIAGNOSE AND TREAT UTERINE DISORDERS.

EXERCISE 20-18

Compare and contrast between each of the following term pairs, referring to your textbook and/or an online dictionary if required.

1. Hysterectomy and myomectomy

   _____

   _____

   _____

2. Hysteroscopy and laparoscopy

   _____

   _____

   _____

3. Myoma and fibroid

   _____

   _____

   _____

11. SHOW HOW WORD PARTS ARE USED TO BUILD WORDS RELATED TO THE REPRODUCTIVE SYSTEMS.

EXERCISE 20-19

Complete the following table by writing the correct word part or meaning in the space provided. Write a word that contains each word part in the Example column.

Word Part	Meaning	Example
1. _____	extreme end	_____
2. fer	_____	_____
3. _____	egg	_____
4. metr/o	_____	_____
5. semin/o	_____	_____
6. test/o	_____	_____
7. _____	ovary	_____
8. rect/o	_____	_____

Making the Connections

The following concept map deals with the female reproductive system. Each pair of terms is linked together by a connecting phrase. Complete the concept map by filling in the appropriate term or phrase. There is one right answer for each term (1, 3, 5, 10). However, there are many correct answers for the connecting phrases.

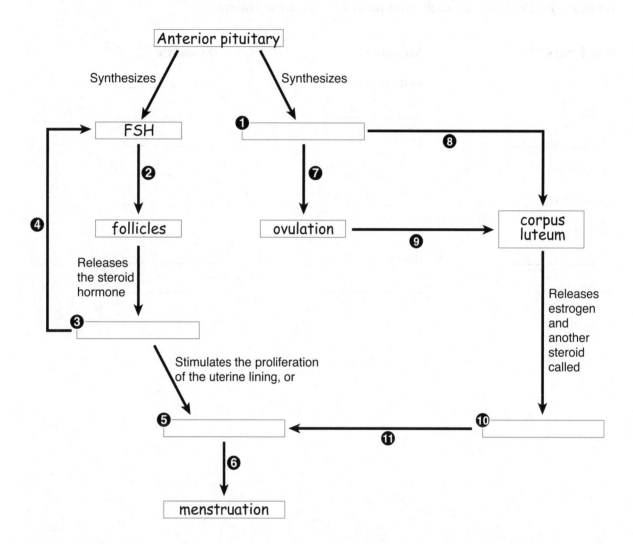

Optional Exercise: Make your own concept map, based on male reproductive anatomy and physiology. Choose your own terms to incorporate into your map, or use the following list: spermatozoon, testosterone, testis, FSH, LH, interstitial cell, epididymis, ductus deferens, seminiferous tubule, sustentacular cell, prostate gland, bulbourethral gland, penis.

Testing Your Knowledge

BUILDING UNDERSTANDING

I. MULTIPLE CHOICE

Select the best answer and write the letter of your choice in the blank.

1. Which of these hormones is secreted by the corpus luteum in
   large amounts?   1. _____
      a. testosterone
      b. progesterone
      c. FSH
      d. LH
2. Which of the following is NOT part of the uterus?   2. _____
      a. fimbriae
      b. cervix
      c. endometrium
      d. corpus
3. In the walls of which structure do spermatozoa develop?   3. _____
      a. prostate gland
      b. penis
      c. seminal vesicles
      d. seminiferous tubules
4. Which of these structures is a gland?   4. _____
      a. corpus cavernosum
      b. seminal vesicle
      c. ductus deferens
      d. epididymis
5. Which of these structures forms the glans penis?   5. _____
      a. corpus spongiosum
      b. corpus cavernosum
      c. pubic symphysis
      d. vas deferens
6. Which of these hormones stimulates ovulation?   6. _____
      a. follicle stimulating hormone
      b. luteinizing hormone
      c. progesterone
      d. testosterone
7. Which of these structures houses the developing ovum?   7. _____
      a. corpus luteum
      b. sustentacular cells
      c. interstitial cells
      d. ovarian follicle

8. Which of the following glands is found in the female?   8. _____
   a. greater vestibular glands
   b. bulbourethral glands
   c. Cowper glands
   d. prostate gland

9. Which of these substances is normally absent from semen?   9. _____
   a. seminal fluid
   b. sugar
   c. a high concentration of hydrogen ions
   d. sperm

II. COMPLETION EXERCISE

Write the word or phrase that correctly completes each sentence.

1. The enzyme-containing cap on the head of a spermatozoon is called the
   _____.

2. The hormone that promotes development of spermatozoa in the male and development of ova in the female is _____.

3. The process of cell division that reduces the chromosome number by half is
   _____.

4. The testes are contained in an external sac called the _____.

5. The main male sex hormone is _____.

6. The pelvic floor in both males and females is called the _____.

7. The hormone that stimulates ovulation is _____.

8. In the male, the tube that carries urine away from the bladder also carries sperm cells. This tube is the _____.

9. A thin, alkaline fluid is secreted into the urethra from the _____.

10. The surgical removal of the foreskin of the penis is called _____.

UNDERSTANDING CONCEPTS

I. TRUE/FALSE

For each question, write T for true or F for false in the blank to the left of each number. If a statement is false, correct it by replacing the underlined term and write the correct statement in the blanks below the question.

_____ 1. A typical semen volume is 2-5 L.

_____

_____ 2. The urethra is contained in the corpus spongiosum of the penis.

_____

_____ 3. The uppermost and widest region of the uterus is the corpus.

_____

_____ 4. Gametes are produced by the process of mitosis.

_____

_____ 5. The pelvic floor is called the peritoneum.

_____

_____ 6. Progesterone levels are highest during the follicular phase of the menstrual cycle.

_____

_____ 7. Progesterone is the first ovarian hormone produced in the menstrual cycle.

_____

_____ 8. A deficiency in luteinizing hormone would result in testosterone deficiency.

_____

II. PRACTICAL APPLICATIONS

Study each discussion. Then write the appropriate word or phrase in the space provided.

➤ **Group A**

1. Ms. J, aged 22, complained of painful menstrual cramps and excessive menstrual flow. The cramps result from excessive contractions of the smooth muscle layer of the uterus, known as the _____.

2. Menstruation is the shedding of the uterine layer called the _____.

3. The physician suggested an anti-inflammatory medication, but Ms. J had previously tried medication to no avail. An alternate approach was tried, in which the passageway between the vagina and the uterus was artificially dilated. The part of the uterus containing this passageway is the _____.

4. The excessive bleeding was also a disturbing symptom. Ultrasound revealed the presence of numerous small, benign uterine tumors. These tumors are called myomas or _____.

5. The tumors were removed by a special instrument that passes through the vagina into the uterine cavity. This instrument is called a(n) _____.

6. Unfortunately, the myomas recurred. Eventually, Ms. J chose to have her uterus removed, a procedure described as a(n) _____.

➤ **Group B**

1. Mr. and Ms. S, both aged 35, had been trying to conceive for two years with no success. Analysis of Mr. S's semen revealed a low concentration of the male gametes, known as _____.

2. Blood tests were performed, revealing a deficiency in the pituitary hormone that acts on sustentacular cells. This hormone is called _____.

3. Conversely, testosterone production was normal. The cells that produce testosterone are called _____.

4. Mr. S's hormone deficiency was successfully treated, and Mr. and Ms. S became the proud parents of triplets. Mr. S went to the clinic shortly after the birth, and his ductus deferens was cut bilaterally. This method of birth control is called a(n) _____.

III. SHORT ESSAYS

1. Discuss changes occurring in the ovary and in the uterus during the follicular phase of the menstrual cycle.

_____
_____
_____

2. Compare and contrast the male and female gametes. Discuss their structure and their production.

_____
_____
_____

CONCEPTUAL THINKING

1. Mr. S is taking synthetic testosterone in order to improve his wrestling performance. To his alarm, he notices that his testicles are shrinking. Explain why this is happening.

   _____

   _____

   _____

2. Compare and contrast the role of FSH in the regulation of the male and female gonad.

   _____

   _____

   _____

Expanding Your Horizons

Have you heard of kamikaze sperm? Based on studies in animals, some animal behavior researchers have hypothesized that semen contains a population of spermatozoa that is capable of destroying spermatozoa from a competing male. A "sperm team" contains blockers, which are misshapen spermatozoa with multiple tails and/or heads. Other sperm, the kamikaze spermatozoa, seek out and destroy spermatozoa from other males. A very small population of egg-getting spermatozoa attempt to fertilize the ovum. Although some aspects of this hypothesis have been challenged, the presence of sperm subpopulations is now well established. You can read more about the kamikaze sperm hypothesis in the scientific articles listed below. The full text of each article is freely available on the internet; do a Web site search for the author and a few words of the title.

- Baker RR, Bellis MA. Elaboration of the Kamikaze sperm hypothesis: a reply to Harcourt. Anim Behav 1989;37:865–867.
- Moore HD, Martin M, Birkhead TR. No evidence for killer sperm or other selective interactions between human spermatozoa in ejaculates of different males in vitro. Proc R Soc Lond B Biol Sci 1999;266:2343–2350.

CHAPTER

21

Development and Heredity

Overview

Pregnancy begins with fertilization of an ovum by a spermatozoon to form a **zygote**. Over the next 38 weeks of **gestation**, the offspring develops first as an **embryo** and then as a **fetus**. During this period, it is nourished and maintained by the **placenta**, formed from tissues of both the mother and the embryo. The placenta secretes a number of hormones, including progesterone, estrogen, human chorionic gonadotropin, human placental lactogen, and relaxin. These hormones induce changes in the uterus and breasts to support the pregnancy and prepare for childbirth and milk production.

Childbirth or **parturition** occurs in four stages, beginning with contractions of the uterus and dilation of the cervix. Subsequent stages include expulsion of the infant, expulsion of the afterbirth, and control of bleeding. Milk production, or **lactation**, is stimulated by the hormones prolactin and oxytocin. Removal of milk from the breasts is the stimulus for continued production.

The scientific study of heredity has advanced with amazing speed in the past 50 years. Nevertheless, many mysteries remain. Gregor Mendel was the first person known to have carried out formal experiments in genetics. He identified independent units of heredity, which he called *factors* and which we now call **genes**.

The chromosomes in the nucleus of each cell are composed of a complex molecule, **DNA**. This material makes up the many thousands of genes that determine a person's traits and are passed on to offspring at the time of fertilization. Genes direct the formation of **enzymes**, which, in turn, make possible all the chemical reactions of metabolism. Some human traits are determined by a single pair of genes (one gene from each parent), but most are controlled by multiple pairs of genes acting together.

Genes may be classified as **dominant** or **recessive**. If one parent contributes a dominant gene, then any offspring who receives that gene will show the trait. Traits carried by recessive genes may remain hidden for generations and be revealed only if they are contributed by both parents.

Addressing the Learning Outcomes

1. DESCRIBE FERTILIZATION AND THE EARLY DEVELOPMENT OF THE FERTILIZED EGG.

EXERCISE 21-1

Write the appropriate term in each blank from the list below.

gestation   zygote   embryo   implantation   morula   fetus   ovum

1. The fertilized egg   _____

2. The developing offspring from the third month until birth   _____

3. The entire period of development in the uterus   _____

4. Attachment of the fertilized egg to the lining of the uterus   _____

5. The developing offspring from implantation until the
   third month   _____

6. The small ball of cells that develops from the zygote   _____

2. DESCRIBE THE STRUCTURE AND FUNCTION OF THE PLACENTA.

Also see Exercise 21-3.

EXERCISE 21-2

Write the appropriate term in each blank from the list below.

chorion   placenta   venous sinuses   chorionic villi
umbilical cord   human placental lactogen   human chorionic gonadotropin
relaxin   endometrium

1. The hormone that loosens the pubic symphysis and softens the
   cervix for parturition   _____

2. A hormone that prepares the breasts for lactation and alters
   maternal metabolism   _____

3. A placental hormone that stimulates progesterone synthesis
   and is detected by pregnancy tests   _____

4. The structure that serves as the organ for nutrition, respiration,
   and excretion for the fetus   _____

5. Projections of the fetal portion of the placenta containing
   fetal capillaries   _____

6. Channels in the placenta containing maternal blood   _____

7. The fetal tissue contributing to the placenta   _____

3. DESCRIBE HOW FETAL CIRCULATION DIFFERS FROM ADULT CIRCULATION.

Also see Exercise 21-5.

EXERCISE 21-3: Fetal Circulation (Text Fig. 21-2)

1. Label the parts of the fetal circulation and placenta.
2. Color the legend boxes red (oxygen-rich blood), blue (oxygen-poor blood), and purple (mixed blood).
3. Color the blood vessels on the diagram based on the oxygen content of the contained blood.

1. _____

2. _____

3. _____

4. _____

5. _____

6. _____

7. _____

8. _____

9. _____

10. _____

11. _____

12. _____

13. _____

14. _____

15. _____

16. _____

17. _____

18. _____

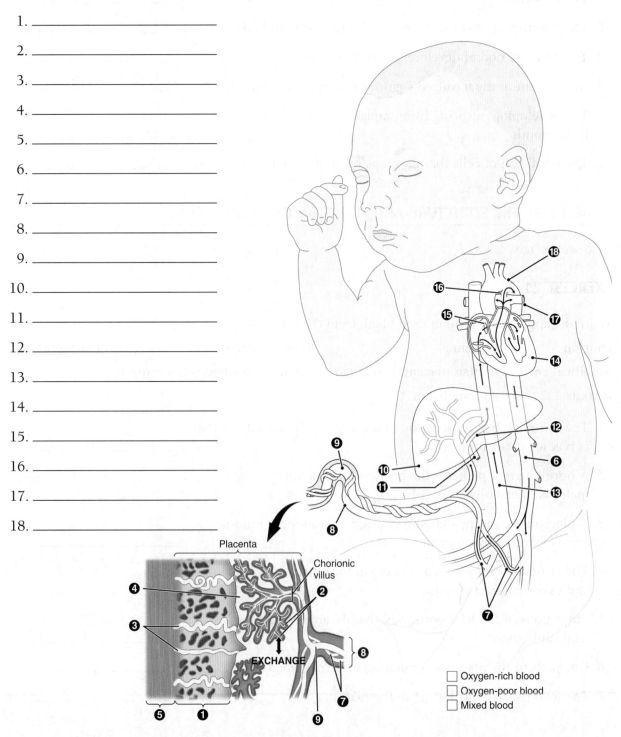

Placenta

Chorionic villus

EXCHANGE

☐ Oxygen-rich blood
☐ Oxygen-poor blood
☐ Mixed blood

4. BRIEFLY DESCRIBE CHANGES THAT OCCUR IN THE EMBRYO, FETUS, AND MOTHER DURING PREGNANCY.

EXERCISE 21-4: Midsagittal Section of a Pregnant Uterus (Text Fig. 21-5)

Write the name of each labeled part on the numbered lines.

1. _____

2. _____

3. _____

4. _____

5. _____

6. _____

7. _____

8. _____

9. _____

10. _____

11. _____

12. _____

13. _____

14. _____

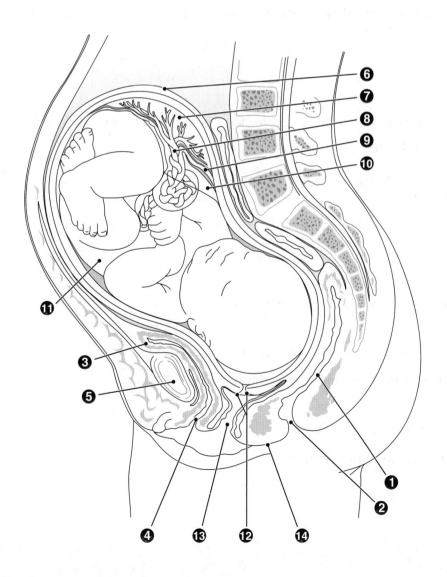

EXERCISE 21-5

Write the appropriate term in each blank from the list below.

vernix caseosa   ultrasonography   ductus venosus   umbilical artery
ductus arteriosus   foramen ovale   amniotic sac   umbilical vein

1. The structure that surrounds the developing offspring and serves as a protective cushion   _____

2. A small vessel joining the pulmonary artery to the descending aorta   _____

3. A small hole in the atrial septum of the fetus   _____

4. The cheeselike material that protects the skin of the fetus   _____

5. A technique commonly used to monitor fetal development   _____

6. The small vessel that enables blood to bypass the liver   _____

7. A major vessel carrying oxygen-rich blood toward the fetus   _____

8. A major vessel carrying oxygen-poor blood away from the fetus   _____

EXERCISE 21-6

Write the appropriate term in each blank from the list below.

oxytocin   prostaglandin   cortisol   negative feedback   positive feedback
first stage   second stage   third stage   fourth stage

1. A fetal hormone that inhibits maternal progesterone secretion and stimulates uterine contractions   _____

2. The hormone that can initiate labor and stimulate milk ejection   _____

3. A substance produced by the myometrium that stimulates uterine contractions   _____

4. The stage of labor that begins when the cervix is completely dilated   _____

5. The stage of labor that ends with the expulsion of the afterbirth   _____

6. The stage of labor in which both the baby and the afterbirth have been expelled   _____

7. The stage of labor during which the cervix dilates   _____

8. The form of feedback regulating oxytocin secretion   _____

5. NAME THE HORMONES ACTIVE IN LACTATION AND DESCRIBE THE ACTION OF EACH.

EXERCISE 21-7

Fill in the blank after each statement—does it apply to prolactin (P) or oxytocin (O)?

1. Produced by the anterior pituitary gland _____

2. Produced by the posterior pituitary gland _____

3. Stimulates milk duct contraction _____

4. Stimulates milk production _____

5. Stimulates the uterine contractions of childbirth. _____

EXERCISE 21-8: Section of the Breast (Text Fig. 21-9)

Write the name of each labeled part on the numbered lines.

1. _____

2. _____

3. _____

4. _____

5. _____

6. _____

7. _____

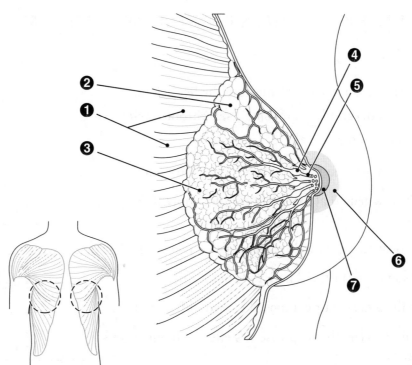

6. CITE THE ADVANTAGES OF BREAST-FEEDING.

EXERCISE 21-9

Briefly summarize four advantages of breast-feeding in the spaces below.

1. _____

2. _____

3. _____

4. _____

7. BRIEFLY DESCRIBE THE MECHANISM OF GENE FUNCTION.

EXERCISE 21-10

Label each of the following statements as true (T) or false (F).

1. Genes are segments of proteins.   _____

2. Genes contain the blueprints to make proteins.   _____

3. Genes are composed of DNA.   _____

4. Genes code for specific traits.   _____

5. Humans have 46 autosomes.   _____

6. Humans have 46 chromosomes.   _____

8. EXPLAIN THE DIFFERENCE BETWEEN DOMINANT AND RECESSIVE GENES.

EXERCISE 21-11

Write the appropriate term in each blank from the list below.

heterozygous   homozygous   autosome   sex chromosome
recessive   dominant   allele

1. One member of a gene pair that controls a specific trait   _____

2. Term describing a gene that expresses its effect only if
   homozygous   _____

3. A gene pair consisting of two dominant or two recessive alleles   _____

4. Any chromosome except the X and Y chromosomes   _____

5. Term describing a gene pair composed of two different alleles   _____

6. Term describing a gene that expresses its effect if homozygous
   or heterozygous   _____

9. COMPARE *PHENOTYPE* AND *GENOTYPE* AND GIVE EXAMPLES OF EACH.

EXERCISE 21-12

Fill in the blank after each statement—does it apply to phenotype (P) or genotype (G)?

1. The genetic makeup of an individual _____

2. The characteristics that can be observed and/or measured _____

3. Eye color _____

4. Homozygous dominant _____

5. Blood type _____

6. Heterozygous _____

10. DESCRIBE WHAT IS MEANT BY A *CARRIER* OF A GENETIC TRAIT.

EXERCISE 21-13

Circle the correct answer.

A carrier of a genetic trait is:

a. an individual heterozygous for a recessive trait.

b. an individual heterozygous for a dominant trait.

c. an individual that shows the symptoms of a disease.

d. an individual homozygous for a recessive trait.

11. DEFINE *MEIOSIS* AND EXPLAIN ITS FUNCTION IN REPRODUCTION.

EXERCISE 21-14

Label each of the following statements as true (T) or false (F).

1. Following meiosis, each reproductive cell contains 46 chromosomes. _____

2. Following meiosis, each reproductive cell contains 23 chromosomes. _____

3. Some reproductive cells contain all of the maternal chromosomes, while other reproductive cells contain all of the paternal chromosomes. _____

4. Each reproductive cell contains a mix of maternal and paternal chromosomes. _____

5. DNA replication always precedes meiosis. _____

6. Meiosis involves two separate cell divisions. _____

7. The paternal and maternal chromosomes separate into separate cells after the second meiotic division. _____

12. EXPLAIN HOW SEX IS DETERMINED IN HUMANS.

EXERCISE 21-15

For each of the following examples, state if the genotype would result in a female phenotype (F) or a male phenotype (M), assuming that development proceeds normally.

1. Union between an X sperm and an X ovum _____

2. Union between a Y sperm and an X ovum _____

13. DESCRIBE WHAT IS MEANT BY THE TERM *SEX-LINKED* AND LIST SEVERAL SEX-LINKED TRAITS.

EXERCISE 21-16

Fill in the blank after each statement—does it refer to sex-linked traits (S) or autosomal (non–sex-linked) traits (A)?

1. A trait carried on the Y chromosome _____

2. A trait carried on the X chromosome _____

3. A trait carried on chromosomes other than the X or Y chromosomes. _____

4. A trait for which males or females can be carriers _____

5. A trait for which only females can be carriers. _____

14. LIST SEVERAL FACTORS THAT MAY INFLUENCE THE EXPRESSION OF A GENE.

EXERCISE 21-17

In the spaces below, list three factors that influence gene expression.

1. _____

2. _____

3. _____

15. REFERRING TO THE CASE STUDY, DESCRIBE THE INHERITANCE OF THE CYSTIC FIBROSIS TRAIT.

EXERCISE 21-18

In the space below, draw a Punnett square for the cross between Ben's parents in regards to the CF trait. You will need to read the case study closely to figure out the genotype of the two parents, and choose your own letters to indicate the different alleles. Then, calculate the probability that they will have a child who is a carrier for the CF trait.

16. SHOW HOW WORD PARTS ARE USED TO BUILD WORDS RELATED TO DEVELOPMENT AND HEREDITY.

EXERCISE 21-19

Complete the following table by writing the correct word part or meaning in the space provided. Write a word that contains each word part in the Example column.

Word Part	Meaning	Example
1. _____	joined	_____
2. toc/o	_____	_____
3. _____	color	_____
4. somat/o	_____	_____
5. phen/o	_____	_____
6. _____	self	_____
7. _____	sharp, acute	_____
8. _____	other, different	_____
9. homo-	_____	_____
10. chori/o	_____	_____

Making the Connections

Map A

The following concept map deals with different aspects of pregnancy, parturition, and lactation. Each pair of terms is linked together by a connecting phrase. Complete the concept map by filling in the appropriate term or phrase. There is one right answer for each term. However, there are many correct answers for the connecting phrases (1, 2, 4, 5, 7, 8, 9).

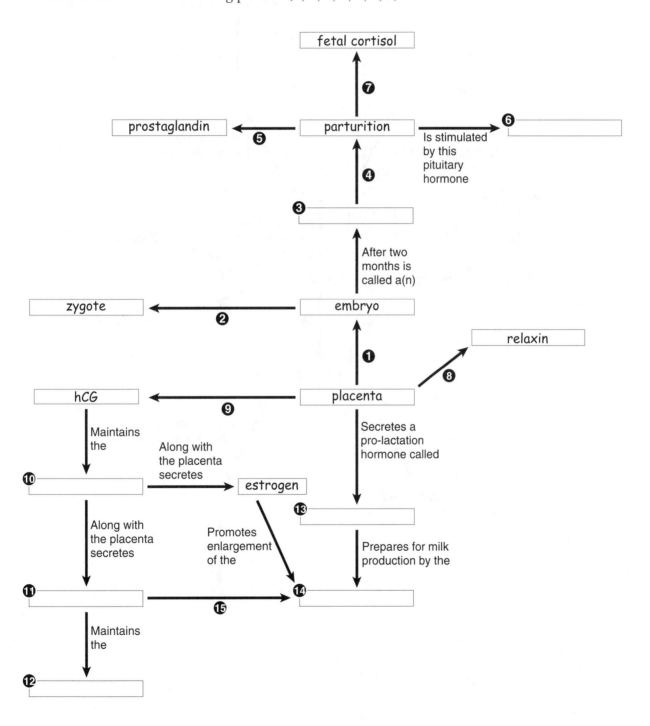

Map B

The following concept map deals with some aspects of heredity. Each pair of terms is linked together by a connecting phrase. Complete the concept map by filling in the appropriate term or phrase. There is one right answer for each term (4 to 6, 11). However, there are many correct answers for the connecting phrases.

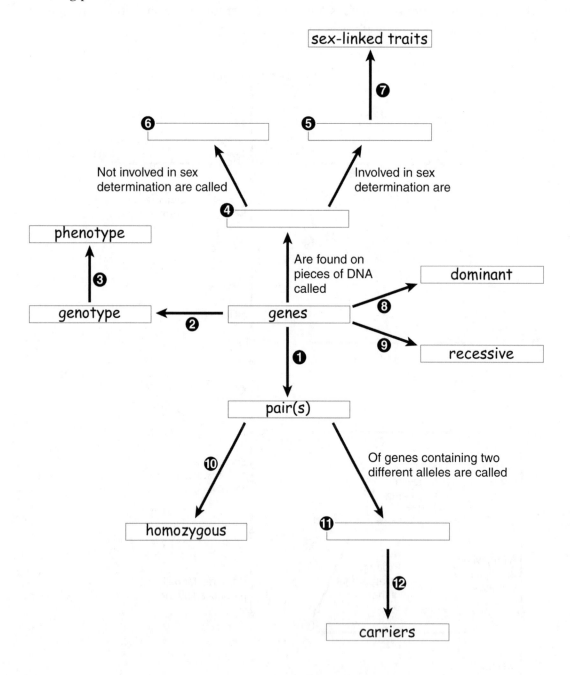

Testing Your Knowledge

BUILDING UNDERSTANDING

I. MULTIPLE CHOICE

Select the best answer and write the letter of your choice in the blank.

1. Which of these substances stimulates contraction of the myometrium?   1. _____
   a. progesterone
   b. estrogen
   c. prolactin
   d. prostaglandin
2. Which two organs are largely bypassed in the fetal circulation?   2. _____
   a. lungs and liver
   b. liver and kidney
   c. lungs and intestine
   d. kidney and intestine
3. What event occurs during the second stage of labor?   3. _____
   a. the onset of contractions
   b. expulsion of the afterbirth
   c. passage of the fetus through the vagina
   d. expulsion of the placenta
4. What determines gender in humans?   4. _____
   a. the number of X chromosomes
   b. the sex chromosome carried by the ovum
   c. the number of autosomes
   d. the sex chromosome carried by the spermatozoon
5. If an imaginary animal has 28 chromosomes per cell, how many
   chromosomes will be found in each spermatozoon?   5. _____
   a. 7
   b. 14
   c. 28
   d. 56
6. Where would you find maternal blood?   6. _____
   a. umbilical cord
   b. chorionic villi
   c. venous sinuses of the placenta
   d. all of the above
7. Which of these is an action of human placental lactogen?   7. _____
   a. maintenance of the corpus luteum
   b. breast development
   c. increased maternal blood glucose levels
   d. growth of the placenta
8. What is a morula?   8. _____
   a. a small ball of cells that implants in the endometrium
   b. the single cell formed by the sperm and ovum
   c. a membrane surrounding the fetus that secretes fluid
   d. a small blood vessel that bypasses the fetal liver

9. Which of these terms describes traits that are determined by more
than one gene pair?   9. _____
      a. sex linked
      b. recessive
      c. multifactorial
      d. dominant

II. COMPLETION EXERCISE

Write the word or phrase that correctly completes each sentence.

1. A surgical cut and repair of the perineum to prevent tearing is called a(n) _____.

2. By the end of the first month of embryonic life, the beginnings of the extremities may be
seen. These are four small swellings called _____.

3. The mammary glands of the female provide nourishment for the newborn through the secretion of milk; this is a process called _____.

4. The stage of labor during which the afterbirth is expelled from the uterus is the
_____.

5. Twins that develop from the same fertilized egg are called _____.

6. The normal site of fertilization is the _____.

7. The clear liquid that flows from the uterus when the mother's "water breaks" is technically
called _____.

8. The larger sex chromosome is called the _____.

9. The number of autosomes in the human genome is _____.

10. The process of cell division that halves the chromosome number is called _____.

11. If the genotype of both parents is Cc, the chance that an offspring will have the genotype CC
is _____.

UNDERSTANDING CONCEPTS

I. TRUE/FALSE

For each question, write T for true or F for false in the blank to the left of each number. If a statement is false, correct it by replacing the underlined term and write the correct statement in the
blanks below the question.

_____1. Ms. J is 7 weeks pregnant. Her uterus contains an embryo.

_____

_____2. The baby is expelled during the fourth stage of labor.

_____

_____3. <u>Fraternal</u> twins are genetically distinct.

_____

_____4. Blood is carried from the placenta to the fetus in the <u>umbilical vein</u>.

_____

_____5. <u>Oxytocin</u> secreted from the fetal adrenal gland may help induce labor.

_____

_____6. The <u>endometrium</u> forms the fetal portion of the placenta.

_____

_____ 7. Sex-linked traits appear almost exclusively in <u>males</u>.

_____

_____ 8. The sex of the offspring is determined by the sex chromosome carried in the <u>spermatozoon.</u>

_____

_____ 9. Carriers for a particular gene are always <u>homozygous</u> for the gene.

_____

_____ 10. A recessive trait is expressed in individuals <u>heterozygous</u> for the recessive gene.

_____

II. PRACTICAL APPLICATIONS

Study each discussion. Then write the appropriate word or phrase in the space provided.

➤ Group A

1. Mr. and Ms. L had been trying to conceive for 2 years. Finally, Ms. L realized her period was late and purchased a pregnancy detection kit. These kits test for the presence of a hormone produced exclusively by embryonic tissues that helps maintain the corpus luteum. This hormone is called _____.

2. The pregnancy test was positive. Six weeks had elapsed since Ms. L's last menstrual period. The gestational age of her new offspring at this time would be _____.

3. During a prenatal appointment 14 weeks later, Ms. L was able to see her future offspring using a technique for visualizing soft tissues without the use of x-rays. This technique is called _____.

4. The pregnancy went smoothly, and the baby was born 5 days early. Ms. L immediately began to breast-feed her infant. The first secretion from her breasts was not milk, but rather _____.

➤ **Group B**

1. Mr. and Ms. J have consulted a genetic counselor. Ms. J is 8 weeks pregnant, and cystic fibrosis runs in both of their families. Cystic fibrosis is a disease in which an individual may carry the disease gene but not have cystic fibrosis. A term to describe this type of trait is _____.

2. Mr. and Ms. J were then screened for the presence of the cystic fibrosis gene. It was determined that both Mr. and Ms. J have the gene even though they do not have cystic fibrosis. For the cystic fibrosis trait, they are both considered to be _____.

3. Ms. J wanted to know if her baby would have cystic fibrosis. The fetus was shown to carry one normal allele and one cystic fibrosis allele. The fact that the alleles are different means that they can be described as _____.

4. The genetic analysis also revealed the presence of two XX chromosomes. The gender of the baby is therefore _____.

III. SHORT ESSAYS

1. Compare and contrast human placental lactogen (hPL) and human chorionic gonadotropin (hCG). Discuss the synthesis and action of each hormone.

_____

_____

_____

_____

2. Describe the site of synthesis and actions of the hormones involved in lactation and preparing the breasts for lactation.

_____

_____

_____

_____

3. Some traits in a population show a range instead of two clearly alternate forms. List some of these traits and explain what causes this variety.

_____

_____

_____

_____

CONCEPTUAL THINKING

1. Trace the path of a blood cell from the placenta to the fetal heart and back to the placenta. Assume that this blood cell passes through the foramen ovale.

   _____

   _____

   _____

   _____

2. Are identical twins identical individuals? Defend your answer, using the terms "genotype" and "phenotype."

   _____

   _____

   _____

3. Describe how each maternal organ changes during pregnancy, and (if relevant) how the change facilitates fetal growth and survival.

   a. heart

   _____

   _____

   b. lungs

   _____

   _____

   c. kidney

   _____

   _____

   d. bladder

   _____

   _____

   e. digestive system

   _____

   _____

Expanding Your Horizons

1. Have you ever wondered why animals can give birth alone, but humans require all sorts of technological equipment? Women rarely give birth alone, even in societies with few technological advances. The difficulties of human birth reflect some of our evolutionary adaptations. For instance, the orientation of the human pelvis facilitates walking upright, but requires the fetus to turn and bend during parturition. You can read more about "The Evolution of Birth" in *Scientific American*.

   • Rosenberg KR, Trevathan WR. Sci Am 2001;285:72–77.

2. The movie *Gattaca* (1997) describes a futuristic world where genetic screening and engineering are the norm. Everyone has a genetic description (including lifespan) available to potential mates, and virtually everyone (except the hero) is genetically engineered. Genetic screening determines one's future on Gattaca, and genetic engineering has essentially abolished independent thought and creativity. Science fiction aside, genetic screening and engineering may soon become a technological reality in our society. What are the implications of genetic screening and engineering? Will a poor genetic outlook affect health insurance coverage and job prospects? Will society genetically engineer away creativity? The articles listed below can provide you with more information about the use and abuse of genetic testing.

   • Hodge JG, Jr. Ethical issues concerning genetic testing and screening in public health. Am J Med Genet 2004;125C: 66–70.
   • Sermon K, Van Steirteghem A, Liebaers I. Preimplantation genetic diagnosis. Lancet 2004;363:1633–1641.